Pruritus in advanced disease

Edited by

Zbigniew Zylicz,
Consultant
Comprehensive Cancer Centre, Nijmegen, The Netherlands
and
Chair of Palliative Care
The Ludwik Rydigier University of Medical Sciences
Bydgoszcz, Poland

Robert Twycross,
Emeritus Clinical Reader in Palliative Medicine
Oxford University
and
Head
WHO Collaborating Centre for Palliative Care
Oxford, UK

and

E. Anthony Jones
Chief of Hepatology
Department of Gastrointestinal and Liver Diseases
Academic Medical Centre
Amsterdam, The Netherlands

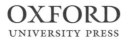

OXFORD
UNIVERSITY PRESS

OXFORD

UNIVERSITY PRESS

Great Clarendon Street, Oxford OX2 6DP

Oxford University Press is a department of the University of Oxford.
It furthers the University's objective of excellence in research, scholarship,
and education by publishing worldwide in

Oxford   New York

Auckland   Bangkok   Buenos Aires   Cape Town   Chennai
Dar es Salaam   Delhi   Hong Kong   Istanbul   Karachi   Kolkata
Kuala Lumpur   Madrid   Melbourne   Mexico City   Mumbai   Nairobi
São Paulo   Shanghai   Taipei   Tokyo   Toronto

Oxford is a registered trade mark of Oxford University Press
in the UK and in certain other countries

Published in the United States by Oxford University Press Inc., New York

A catalogue record for this title is available from the British Library

ISBN 0 19 852510 9

10 9 8 7 6 5 4 3 2 1

Typeset by Cepha Imaging Pvt Ltd
Printed in Great Britain
on acid-free paper by
Ashford Colour Press Ltd, Gosport, Hampshire

Preface

In 2000, a multispecialty seminar on pruritus was held in Oxford (UK) under the auspices of the Oxford International Centre for Palliative Care. We soon realized how little most of us knew about pruritus, working separately in our individual specialties, and how much we could gain from each other. The seminar participants agreed to work on a book to integrate the knowledge from the different specialties and so provide guidance to other clinicians when confronted with this problem.

Pruritus is a prevalent symptom in many skin conditions. However, much less is known about pruritus without primary skin disease—the so-called *pruritus sine materiae*. This problem occurs in most medical specialties, notably internal medicine, haematology, oncology, hepatology, nephrology, anaesthesiology, immunology, and psychiatry. Specialists from these disciplines each see few patients with severe pruritus and therefore have only a limited possibility to learn from their experience. Their approach is usually through diagnosing and controlling the underlying systemic disease. When asked for an opinion, the dermatologist with his or her excellent visual pattern recognition capabilities can seldom provide a clue.

Pruritus or itch may be a symptom of a systemic disease, but it also may be the result of poor hygiene or insect bite. Most of the patients suffering from severe generalized pruritus will tell their doctor, 'It's much worse than pain' or 'I wish it was pain; then at least there would be a remedy for it.' Thus, the aim of this book is to build a bridge of knowledge and evidence between the various specialties.

Inevitably, the book will share both the strengths and weaknesses of most multiauthor books. It gains by having the opinions of physicians with widely different clinical backgrounds but, in some places, will seem disjointed in style and content. Occasionally, there may be contradictions. Even so, we believe that the discerning reader will find much practical advice in its pages and will be further stimulated by the different emphases of the various authors.

ZZ   *June 2003*
RT
EAJ

Contents

Abbreviations

5-HT	5-hydroxytryptamine
ADP	adenosine diphosphate
b.d.	*bis die* (twice daily); alternatively b.i.d.
CAPD	continuous ambulatory peritoneal dialysis
CGRP	calcitonin gene-related peptide
CMH	C-fibre mechano-heat nociceptors
CNS	central nervous system
CRH	corticotropin-releasing hormone
EEG	electroencephalography
EMLA	eutectic mixture of local anaesthetics (cream)
EPPER	eosinophilic, polymorphic, and pruritic eruption associated with radiotherapy
fMRI	functional magnetic resonance imaging
fPET	functional positron emission tomography
GABA-A	gamma-aminobutyric acid-A
HES	hydroxyethyl starch
IL-2	interleukin 2
IV	intravenous
IVLEN	inflammatory linear verrucous epidermal naevus
MHP	monosymptomatic hypochondriacal psychosis
m-PTH	mid-region PTH
NGF	nerve growth factor
NSAIDs	nonsteroidal anti-inflammatory drugs
NT	neurotensin
NT_4	neurotrophin 4

OCD	obsessive–compulsive disorder
o.n.	*omni nocte* (at bedtime)
PAR	proteinase-activated receptors
PCA	patient-controlled analgesia
PgE$_2$	prostaglandin E$_2$
p.r.n.	*pro re nata*, as needed
PTH	parathyroid hormone
PUVA	psoralen + ultraviolet A (therapy)
PVDF	polyvinylidene fluoride
q.d.s.	*quarter die sumendus* (four times daily)
SC	subcutaneous
SP	substance P
SSRI	selective serotonin reuptake inhibitors
t.d.s.	*ter die sumendus* (three times a day)
TNFα	tumour necrosis factor alpha
TRK-A	thyrosine receptor kinase A
UVB	ultraviolet B
VAS	visual analogue scale
VMpo	ventromedial thalamic nucleus
VR$_1$	vanilloid receptor 1

Contributors

Nora V. Bergasa
Division of Digestive and Liver Diseases, College of Physicians and Surgeons of Columbia University, New York, USA

Petra Eland de Kok
Department of Dermatology, University Medical Centre Utrecht, Utrecht, The Netherlands

Hermann O. Handwerker
Department of Physiology and Experimental Pathophysiology, University of Erlangen/Nürnberg, Erlangen, Germany

E. Anthony Jones
Department of Gastrointestinal and Liver Diseases, Academic Medical Center, Amsterdam, The Netherlands

John Y. Koo
UCSF Medical Center, Psoriasis and Skin Treatment Center, Department of Dermatology, San Francisco, California, USA

Małgorzata Krajnik
Department of Palliative Care, The Ludwik Rydygier University of Medical Sciences, Bydgoszcz, Poland

Roger S. Lo
UCLA Medical Center, Division of Dermatology, Los Angeles, California, USA

Hugo Molenaar
Department of Electronics, Academic Medical Center, Amsterdam, The Netherlands

Harmieke van Os-Medendorp
Department of Dermatology, University Medical Centre Utrecht, Utrecht, The Netherlands

Martin Schmelz
Department of Anesthesiology Mannheim, University of Heidelberg, Mannheim, Germany

Jacek C. Szepietowski
Department of Dermatology, Venereology, and Allergology, University of Medicine, Wrocław, Poland

Robert Twycross
Emeritus Clinical Reader in Palliative Medicine, Oxford University, Oxford, UK

Zbigniew Zylicz
Comprehensive Cancer Centre, Nijmegen, The Netherlands, and Department of Palliative Care, The Ludwik Rydygier University of Medical Sciences, Bydgoszcz, Poland

An introduction to pruritus

Zbigniew Zylicz

Pruritus and evolution

We all grow up with pain but, because we are afraid of it, we learn to avoid it. In fact the whole of our life is impregnated with this fear. In the course of evolution, humans gained insights that made them more vulnerable not only to physical, but also psychological and spiritual pain.[1] It is different with pruritus. While pain has become more important, pruritus has become less so. During the early stages of evolution, the whole bodies of our ancestors were covered with thick fur. Pruritus helped to identify unwanted parasites and their irritating excrements, and other dirt. Pruritus initiated scratching, which was necessary to keep the fur clean. Scratching also increases skin blood circulation and helps to clear skin inflammation. It is tempting to speculate that, when hominid apes came down from the trees and started to walk in the upright position, they lost the ability to reach every part of their backs. Perhaps after that they formed clans because they needed each other for scratching backs. Who knows? Perhaps pruritus played an important and underestimated role in the development and socialization of the hominids.

Meaning of pruritus

At the present time, human beings are more pain- than pruritus-oriented. Only about 5% of the C-fibres entering the dorsal horn are sensitive to itch stimuli.[2] Other C-fibres are used for conduction of pain and mechano- and thermo-receptive stimuli. However, in dogs this representation is higher as pruritus plays an important role in the maintenance of health.[3, 4] For human beings, who have lost most of their body hair, pruritus has a more limited signalling function. It still warns about the presence of parasites and insects, their toxins and excrements (e.g. scabies), but also warns about the toxic effects of some chemicals (contact dermatitis) and sunlight (sunburn). We learn how to avoid such chemicals in order to prevent pruritus.

Definition

Pruritus is an unpleasant sensation that provokes the desire to scratch.[5] But, like many 'working' definitions, this is not fully correct. Pruritus is not necessarily unpleasant. Some people say that they experience pleasure when scratching. At least at the beginning. Because pain inhibits pruritic impulses in the spinal cord (see Chapter 2), many patients scratch until they cause pain, in order to experience relief from pruritus. However, many others do experience severe pruritus and pain at the same time, and they have little desire to scratch, knowing well that relief will not ensue.

Mucous membranes and pruritus

Pruritus can affect not only the skin. It may also affect all mucous membranes. Conjunctival pruritus will usually provoke tear production, rubbing and fluttering of the eyelids, but not scratching. Vaginal discharge and inflammation may cause pruritus vulvae.[6]

Terminology

Should we use word *pruritus* or *itch*? It would be logical to make a choice and to use only one of them, namely, *pruritus*. Pruritus is a Latin word and is well understood in many languages. However, this word also has its limitations. You may say 'something is the cause of my pruritus', but you will always say, 'my leg is itching'. Both words mean the same and will be used interchangeably in this book. For other terms used in this book please see Table 1.1.

Prevalence

The prevalence of pruritus is difficult to estimate, partly because pruritus is a subjective experience. Mild-to-moderate pruritus is experienced by many, otherwise healthy people. The prevalence of pruritus increases with age.[7] It is said that 60–80% of old people suffer from occasional pruritus, but it is obvious that not all suffer from senile pruritus, which is a distinct

Table 1.1 Terminology

Pruritus or itch	An unpleasant sensation that provokes the desire to scratch
Pruritogens	Substances that cause pruritus, usually by acting at the pruritus receptors localized at the C-nerve endings. Counterparts of algogens
Antipruritics	Drugs and substances that may help to relieve pruritus
Pruritoceptive pruritus	Pruritus that results from stimulation of specific receptors on a subset of mucocutaneous C-fibres
Pruritic mediators	Substances involved in transmission of pruritus in the second- and third-order neurons
Neuropathic pruritus	Pruritus experienced in an area of changed sensibility. It is usually caused by an anatomical change within the nervous system (e.g. nerve damage or brain tumour)
Neurogenic pruritus	Pruritus caused by pruritic mediators interfering with itch transmission and the functioning of the nervous system
Alloknesis	Touch-evoked pruritus; analogous to allodynia
Hyperknesis	Increased itch response to pruritogens, e.g. histamine iontophoresis
Pruralgia	Pruritus experienced together with pain
Dysaesthesia	An unpleasant abnormal sensation, whether spontaneous or evoked
Painful polyneuropathy	Neuropathy affecting multiple peripheral sensory nerves, e.g. when the cause is systemic
Mononeuropathy	Neuropathy affecting one single nerve, e.g. nerve entrapment

entity.[8] Atopic dermatitis, the most common pruritic skin disease, is more prevalent in children.[9, 10] In some conditions pruritus is rare and does not contribute to the diagnosis, for example, in solid tumours. In other conditions it is very frequent and nearly obligatory for diagnosis, for example, in Sezary syndrome.[11] In advanced diseases, as seen in palliative care units, the prevalence of severe pruritus is low and the causes are diverse. This makes specific research difficult, if not impossible. Many patients may have other symptoms, such as pain, nausea, and constipation, and these symptoms may 'suppress' the reporting of pruritus. On the other hand, pain, which is very common in advanced diseases, may suppress pruritus (see Chapter 2).

There are many diseases that may be accompanied by pruritus, mainly skin diseases (Table 1.2, modified from reference 12). These diseases may have an acute character, for example, urticaria, which may spontaneously remit when the contact with the initiating factor ceases. Urticaria is usually ascribed to the release of histamine from the mast cells. This type of reaction may be called 'pruritoceptive' itch, as it is the normal reaction to skin infestation. However, when the contact with pruritogens is prolonged, or the host is constitutionally susceptible to them, pruritus may become chronic and may be more and more independent of the peripheral stimulation, for example, atopic dermatitis. This situation depends on central sensitization, which will be discussed later.

However, some skin diseases associated with pruritus may be the consequence of an internal disorder (Table 1.3). Successful treatment of the underlying condition normally relieves the accompanying pruritus. However, in many cases, a symptomatic approach may be the only therapeutic option.

Classification

Pruritus can be peripheral (pruritoceptive) in origin or it may be the result of anatomical and/or functional changes in the nerves transmitting these impulses.[13] These changes may be peripheral (peripheral neuropathy) or central (brain tumour or abscess). Additionally, central causes of itch may be neurogenic or psychogenic. Essential or idiopathic pruritus is pruritus of unknown origin.

Pruritoceptive pruritus

Pruritoceptive pruritus may originate in the skin or mucous membranes and is a result of activation of specific receptors at the specialized C-fibre endings.[14] The impulses are conveyed to the dorsal horns of the spinal cord and, after synapsing there, they are conveyed to the central nervous system. The nerve endings are sensitive to histamine, which may be released from the mast cells under the influence of many substances called pruritogens. Pruritoceptive pruritus may be acute, for example, acute urticaria, or chronic, for example, atopic dermatitis. Acute pruritoceptive

Table 1.2 Skin conditions that may be associated with troublesome pruritus. (Modified from ref. 12)

Infestation	*Infections*
Insect bites, papular urticaria	Varicella
Pediculosis	Dermatophytosis
Scabies and other mites	Bacterial folliculitis
Schistosomal cercarial dermatitis (swimmer's itch)	Candidal folliculitis
Inflammatory	Pityrosporum folliculitis
Atopic dermatitis	Impetigo
Allergic and irritant contact dermatitis	*Hereditary or congenital*
Urticaria	Darier–White disease (keratosis follicularis)
Dermatitis herpetiformis	Hailey–Hailey disease (benign familial pemphigus)
Drug hypersensitivity	Inflammatory linear verrucous epidermal naevus (IVLEN)
Psoriasis	*Neoplastic*
Pemphigoid	Mycosis fungoides (cutaneous T-cell lymphoma)
Mastocytosis	Paraneoplastic pruritus
Lichen simplex chronicus	
Prurigo nodularis (can also be secondary to scratching)	
Lichen planus (not always)	
Miliaria	

Table 1.2 Skin conditions that may be associated with troublesome pruritus. (Modified from ref. 12) (*contd*)

Miscellaneous

Xerosis	Fox–Fordyce disease (apocrine miliaria)
Asteatotic eczema, eczema craquele	Exanthematous drug eruptions
'Winter itch'	Aquagenic pruritus
Dermographism and other forms of physical urticaria	Aerogenic pruritus (atmoknesis)
Pityriasis rosea	Anogenital pruritus
Pityriasis rubra pilaris	Sunburn
Parapsoriasis	Exfoliative dermatitis
Grover's disease (transient acantholytic disease)	Senile pruritus
Persistent acantholytic dermatosis	Contact pruritus
Pruritic urticarial papules and plaques of pregnancy	Cholinergic pruritus
Folliculitis	Adrenergic pruritus
Perforating folliculitis	Flushing
Acquired perforating dermatosis	Lichen amyloidosis
Eosinophilic pustular folliculitis	Macular cutaneous amyloidosis (notalgia paraesthetica)
Infundibulofolliculitis	'Itchy red bump disease' (prurigo simplex subacuta)

Table 1.3 Systemic non-skin diseases that may be accompanied by pruritus

Chronic renal failure (uraemic pruritus)
Polycythemia rubra vera
Cholestasis
Hodgkin's lymphoma
Iron deficiency anaemia
Malignant carcinoid
Multiple myeloma
Solid tumours (paraneoplastic)
Scleroderma
Hyperthyroidism
Anorexia nervosa

Systemic infection
   HIV infection
   Schistosomiasis
   Onchocerciasis (river blindness)
   Ascariasis
   Hookworm
   Trichinosis
   Parvovirus B19

pruritus often responds to H_1-antihistamines.[15, 16] However, the more chronic pruritus is, the more central sensitization is present. In these cases, response to H_1-antihistamines may decrease or even disappear.

Neuropathic pruritus

Neuropathic pruritus (see Chapter 10), similarly to neuropathic pain, occurs in areas of skin with changed sensibility. It may originate at any point along the afferent pathway as a result of damage and to other secondary changes in that pathway. Neuropathic pruritus and pain may result from herpetic infection of a peripheral nerve[17] or pruritus alone from sensory nerve entrapment involving posterior rami of T2–T6, a condition called notalgia paraesthetica.[18] Severe unilateral neuropathic pruritus can result from cerebral tumour, abscess, or thrombosis.[18–22] These conditions are only rarely reversible and are not H_1-antihistamine-responsive.

Neurogenic pruritus

Neurogenic pruritus originates centrally in spinal cord or brain, and is caused by accumulation of endogenous or exogenous toxins. These toxins may function as pruritus mediators. As an example, pruritus accompanying cholestasis is probably due to retention or abnormal production of the endogenous opioid agonists.[23] Similar symptoms may be evoked by exogenous opioids administered spinally.[24,25] The site of action is probably localized in medullary dorsal horn.[25] This type of pruritus resolves after removing the toxic factor or antagonizing it at the receptor site. Neurogenic pruritus is histamine-independent and H_1-antihistamines do not relieve it.

Continuous peripheral neural discharge may cause central sensitization.[26,27] On occasion this may result in severe neurogenic pruritus. As we do not understand fully the phenomenon of central sensitization, we have only limited means to treat it pharmacologically. Recently, it has been postulated that glial cells in the central nervous system may play an important role in sensitization and in maintaining this condition, sometimes for life.[28] It seems possible that, in the future, we will understand central sensitization better. It is also possible that we will be able to investigate existing drugs as potential antipruritics. However, it is improbable that new drugs specifically designed and developed for this purpose will be developed. Development costs are too expensive in relation to the small and heterogeneous group of patients who might benefit from such drugs.

Psychogenic pruritus

Psychogenic pruritus is a separate category (see Chapter 11). There is usually no specific identifiable cause and antipruritic drugs, except antidepressants, are generally ineffective. The apparent favourable effect of H_1-antihistamines probably depends on their sedative properties, and not on any specific effect on pruritus.[16] However, psychotherapy and psychotropic drugs that relieve tension, depression, and anxiety may help psychogenic pruritus. Humans are sensitive to suggestion and, occasionally, psychogenic pruritus may occur in several or many individuals concurrently or sequentially.[29] Psychogenic pruritus may be associated with certain psychiatric disorders.

Conclusions

• While pain can be meaningful to humans, pruritus is not.
• Pruritus and itch have the same meaning.

- Pain frequently suppresses pruritus in the spinal cord. However, sometimes pain and pruritus are experienced simultaneously.
- Pruritus is an unpleasant feeling that provokes scratching.
- Pruritus can be divided into pruritoceptive, neurogenic, neuropathic, and psychogenic.
- Psychogenic pruritus is a specific condition. The diagnosis is not made only by simple exclusion of other known causes of pruritus.

References

1. Saunders C. (1988). Spiritual pain. *J Palliat Care* **4**:29–32.
2. Schmelz M, Michael K, Weidner C, Schmidt R, Torebjörk HE, Handwerker HO. (2000). Which nerve fibers mediate the axon reflex flare in human skin? *Neuroreport* **11**:645–8.
3. Doody GM. (1990). Non-specific pruritus in dogs. *Vet Rec* **126**:273–4.
4. Anonymous. (1981). Pruritus in dogs. *Mod Vet Pract* **62**:651–2.
5. Rothman S. (1941). Physiology of itching. *Physiol Rev* **21**:357–81.
6. Chan L. (1989). Investigation and treatment of vaginal discharge and pruritus vulvae. *Singapore Med J* **30**:471–2.
7. Rea JN, Newhouse ML, Halil T. (1976). Skin disease in Lambeth. A community study of prevalence and use of medical care. *Br J Prev Soc Med* **30**:107–14.
8. Kelly R. (1977). Dermatoses in geriatric patients. *Aust Fam Physician* **6**:36–44.
9. Leung AK, Wong BE, Chan PY, Cho HY. (1998). Pruritus in children. *J R Soc Health* **118**:280–6.
10. Taylor B, Wadsworth J, Wadsworth M, Peckham C. (1984). Changes in the reported prevalence of childhood eczema since the 1939–45 war. *Lancet* **2**:1255–7.
11. Kantor AF, Curtis RE, Vonderheid EC, van Scott EJ, Fraumeni JF Jr. (1989). Risk of second malignancy after cutaneous T-cell lymphoma. *Cancer* **63**:1612–15.
12. Bernhard JD. (1994). Pruritus in skin diseases. In: JD Bernhard (ed.), *Itch. Mechanisms and management of pruritus*, New York: McGraw-Hill, pp. 37–67.
13. Twycross R, Greaves MW, Handwerker H, *et al.* (2003). Itch: scratching more than the surface. *QJM* **96**:7–26.
14. Schmelz M, Schmidt R, Bickel A, Handwerker HO, Torebjörk HE. (1997). Specific C-receptors for itch in human skin. *J Neurosci* **17**:8003–8.
15. Arnold AJ, Simpson JG, Jones HE, Ahmed AR. (1979). Suppression of histamine-induced pruritus by hydroxyzine and various neuroleptics. *J Am Acad Dermatol* **1**:509–12.
16. Krause L, Shuster S. (1983). Mechanism of action of antipruritic drugs. *Br Med J (Clin Res Ed)* **287**:1199–200.

17. Oaklander AL, Cohen SP, Raju SV. (2002). Intractable postherpetic itch and cutaneous deafferentation after facial shingles. *Pain* **96**:9–12.

18. Layton AM, Cotterill JA. (1991). Notalgia paraesthetica—report of three cases and their treatment. *Clin Exp Dermatol* **16**:197–8.

19. Andreev VC, Petkov I. (1975). Skin manifestations associated with tumours of the brain. *Br J Dermatol* **92**:675–8.

20. King CA, Huff FJ, Jorizzo JL. (1982). Unilateral neurogenic pruritus: paroxysmal itching associated with central nervous system lesions. *Ann Intern Med* **97**:222–3.

21. Massey EW. (1984). Unilateral neurogenic pruritus following stroke. *Stroke* **15**:901–3.

22. Sandroni P. (2002). Central neuropathic itch: a new treatment option? *Neurology* **59**:778.

23. Jones EA, Bergasa NV. (1999). The pruritus of cholestasis. *Hepatology* **29**:1003–6.

24. Ballantyne JC, Loach AB, Carr DB. (1988). Itching after epidural and spinal opiates. *Pain* **33**:149–60.

25. Thomas DA, Williams GM, Iwata K, Kenshalo DR Jr, Dubner R. (1993). The medullary dorsal horn. A site of action of morphine in producing facial scratching in monkeys. *Anesthesiology* **79**:548–54.

26. Kessler M, Moneret-Vautrin DA, Cao-Huu T, Mariot A, Chanliau J. (1992). Dialysis pruritus and sensitization. *Nephron* **60**:241.

27. Alteras I, Grunwald M. (1981). The possible role of fungal sensitization in the pathogenesis of generalized essential pruritus. *Mykosen* **24**:107–10.

28. Watkins LR, Milligan ED, Maier SF. (2001). Spinal cord glia: new players in pain. *Pain* **93**:201–5.

29. Robinson P, Szewczyk M, Haddy L, Jones P, Harvey W. (1984). Outbreak of itching and rash. Epidemic hysteria in an elementary school. *Arch Intern Med* **144**:1959–62.

2

Neurophysiology

Martin Schmelz and
Hermann O. Handwerker

Itch and pain pathways

In the past, low level activation of nociceptors was thought to induce pruritus, and a higher discharge frequency to induce pain.[1] Consistent with this theory was the observation that the intradermal application of high concentrations of pruritogens, e.g. histamine, may cause pain. On the other hand, application of low concentrations of algogens does not cause itch, just less intense pain. Further, intraneural electrical microstimulation of human afferent nerves induces either pain or, less commonly, pruritus. Increasing the stimulation frequency increases the intensity of pain or itch but no switch from pruritus to pain is observed. Likewise, a decrease of stimulation frequency at a site, where pain has been elicited, decreases the magnitude of pain; at no point does it induce itch.[2]

Firing frequency in nociceptors cannot therefore account for the differentiation between pain and itch. It must be assumed that pruritogens preferentially excite a distinct subgroup of C-fibres, which give rise to itch. Such C-fibres have been discovered among mechano-insensitive C-nociceptors which respond to histamine iontophoresis in parallel to the itch ratings of subjects (Fig. 2.1).[3] In contrast, the most common type of C-fibres, mechano-heat nociceptors (CMH or polymodal nociceptors) are either insensitive to histamine or only weakly activated by it.[4, 5] They cannot account for the prolonged itch induced by the intradermal application of histamine.

The histamine-sensitive or 'itch' fibres are characterized by:

- low conduction velocity
- large innervation territories

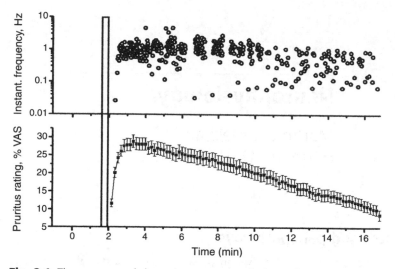

Fig. 2.1 The upper panel shows instantaneous discharge frequency of a mechano- and heat-insensitive C-fibre (CMiHi) in the superficial peroneal nerve following histamine iontophoresis (20 mC; marked as open box in the diagram). The unit was not spontaneously active before histamine application, but continued to fire for about 15 minutes after application (not shown in the diagram). The lower panel shows average pruritus magnitude ratings of a group of 21 healthy volunteers, after an identical histamine stimulus. Ratings at 10 second intervals on a visual analogue scale (VAS) with the end-points 'no itch' → 'unbearable itch'. Bars: means ± SEM.[3]

- mechanical unresponsiveness
- high transcutaneous electrical thresholds.

In line with the large innervation territories of these fibres, two point discrimination for histamine-induced itch is poor (15 cm in the upper arm).[6]

The relative prevalence of the different fibre types among the C-fibres has been estimated from recordings in the superficial peroneal nerve.[7] About 80% are polymodal nociceptors, which respond to mechanical, heat and chemical stimuli. The remaining 20% do not respond to mechanical stimulation. These fibres are mainly 'silent' or 'sleeping' nociceptors.[8–12] They are activated by chemical stimuli,[13] and can be sensitized to mechanical stimulation in the presence of inflammation.[13, 14] In addition, there is a subset of non-nociceptive fibres which have a strong and

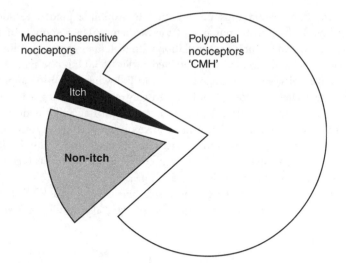

Fig. 2.2 Relative proportion of mechano-responsive and mechano-insensitive unmyelinated C-fibres in human skin nerves. About 20% of the C-fibres are mechano-insensitive. Itch units are found only among these mechano-insensitive fibres.

sustained response to histamine. They comprise about 20% of the mechano-heat-insensitive class of C-fibres, i.e. 4-5% of all C-fibres (Fig. 2.2).

Primary afferent 'itch-neurons'

Only a few mediators can induce histamine-independent pruritus. Prostaglandins enhance histamine-induced itch[15, 16] but also act directly as pruritogens in the conjunctiva.[16, 17] and in human skin when applied via microdialysis.[18] Serotonin injected intradermally has been found to elicit mostly pain, but also a weak itch sensation.[19] Recent findings suggest that the peripheral effect of serotonin may be partly due to release of histamine from mast cells.[20] The role of serotonin in the pathogenesis of itch is unclear. It might be involved in pruritus in policythaemia vera.[19]

An intra-dermal injection of acetylcholine is pruritogenic in atopic subjects, but induces pain in non-atopic subjects.[21] This finding may explain why many atopic patients experience itch when sweating. In normal skin the relative potency of the best known pruritogens is histamine $\gg$ prostaglandin E_2 > acetylcholine = serotonin. Bradykinin or capsaicin application usually induces pain only. Primary afferent neurons mediating itch sensations would thus be expected to exhibit a graded response according to the pruritic potency of the mediators. The responses of the different types of C-fibres to stimulation with histamine, prostaglandin E_2, acetylcholine, and capsaicin are depicted in Fig. 2.3. Only the mechano-insensitive units, with prolonged activation following histamine application were excited by prostaglandin E_2. In contrast, long-lasting activation of mechano-responsive units by histamine or by prostaglandin E_2 does not occur. Likewise, all the mechano-insensitive fibres, which were unresponsive to histamine, were also unresponsive to prostaglandin E_2 application. Thus, the response pattern of the histamine-responsive itch units is consistent with the observed pruritic effects of PgE_2.

Intradermal injection of PgE_2 produces only a weak weal.[22, 23] It has been claimed that intradermal injection of PgE_2 also results in a small

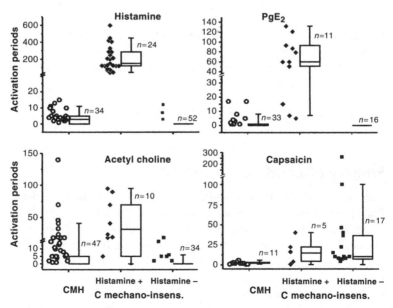

Fig. 2.3 Intensity of chemically induced activation of different classes of C-nociceptors (mechano-heat responsive fibres 'CMH' = polymodal nociceptors; histamine-responsive ('Histamine +') and histamine-non-responsive ('Histamine −') mechano-insensitive fibres (C mechano-insens.). The units were stimulated with histamine (iontophoresis; 20 mC), prostaglandin E_2 (PgE_2; 10^{-5} M, 20 µl injection), acetylcholine (iontophoresis; 60 mC), or capsaicin (0.1%, 20 µl injection).

amount of protein extravasation.[24, 25] However, with a more refined technique, namely the dermal application of PgE_2 via microdialysis combined with measurement of local protein extravasation and local blood flow, it has been shown that PgE_2 does not increase protein extravasation, even at a concentration of $10^{-4}M$, but causes mild itch and pronounced vasodilation. These findings support the notion of an histamine-independent pruritogenic action of PgE_2, since histamine provokes protein extravasation at lower concentrations than that required for itch induction.[26] Thus, one can conclude that the terminals of itch units contain membrane receptors for prostaglandins, and possibly other agents, in addition to those for histamine.

In the light of the pruritogenic effects of PgE_2, activation of histamine-responsive chemoreceptors by this mediator provides a strong argument for a fairly specific neuronal system for itch, separate from the pain pathway. However, the histamine-responsive fibres are also excited by at least one specific algogen, namely capsaicin. The observation that capsaicin induces not only pain but also activates itch, may be explained by an inhibition of itch by pain in the central nervous system (see Fig. 2.5 left panel). To distinguish psychochemical specificity (which apparently does not exist) from selective projection into separate central pathways, itch neurons have been termed 'itch selective'.[27] The activation of itch neurons by algogens like capsaicin does not contradict a 'labeled line' for itch suggested by the discovery of histamine-sensitive central neurons.[28]

In summary, the pruritogenic potency of inflammatory mediators is characterized by their ability to activate histamine-sensitive mechano-insensitive C-fibres. However, concomitant activation of mechano-sensitive and mechano-insensitive histamine-unresponsive nociceptors will decrease itch and increase pain. Thus, itch sensation is based on both activity in the itch pathway and a low level of activity in the pain pathway.

Specific spinal itch-neurons

The concept of dedicated itch neurons has now been complemented and extended by recordings from the cat spinal cord. A specific class of dorsal horn neurons projecting to the thalamus has been demonstrated, which responds strongly to histamine administered to skin by iontophoresis . The time course of these responses was similar to that of itch in humans and matched the responses of the peripheral C-itch fibres (see Fig. 2.1). These units were also unresponsive to mechanical stimulation and differed from the non-histamine-sensitive nociceptive units in lamina I of the spinal cord. In addition, their axons had a lower conduction velocity and anatomically distinct projections to the thalamus. Thus, the combination of dedicated peripheral and central neurons that have a unique response pattern to pruritogenic mediators and anatomically distinct projections to the thalamus, provide the basis for a specific neuronal pathway for itch.

Central itch processing

The itch-selective units in lamina I of the spinal cord form a distinct pathway projecting to the posterior part of the ventromedial thalamic nucleus (VMpo), which projects to the dorsal insular cortex[29] a region which has been shown to be involved in a variety of interoceptive modalities like thermoception, visceral sensations, thirst and hunger. The supraspinal processing of itch and its corresponding scratch response have recently been investigated in man by functional positron emission tomography (fPET). Induction of itch by intradermal histamine injections and histamine skin prick elicit co-activation of the anterior cingulate cortex, supplementary motor area and inferior parietal lobe with left hemisphere predominance.[30–32] The significant co-activation of the motor area supports the clinical observation that itch is inherently linked to a desire to scratch. The multiple activated sites in the brain after itch induction argue against the existence of a single itch centre and reflect the multidimensionality of itch. The central neuropatho-physiology is very similar for pain and itch and, indeed, a broad overlap of activated brain areas is evident for pain and itch. However, subtle differences in the activation pattern between itch and pain have been described, such as (with itch) a lack of secondary somatosensory cortex activation of the parietal operculum and left hemispheric dominance.

By use of functional magnetic resonance imaging (fMRI) and histamine iontophoresis to provoke itch in human volunteers, it has been shown that several forebrain regions (Brodman areas 10, 21, 22, 40) and also the cerebellum are activated by itch.[14] The increasing availability of fMRI and further technical development of central imaging techniques will lead to closer insights into the central representation of itch, so that recordings in patients with itch become realistic, as in the field of pain.

Itch mediators

Histamine, substance P and other neuropeptides

Histamine has been a widely used pruritogen in experimental settings.[33] It has been shown that most experimental itch stimuli act indirectly via release of histamine from cutaneous mast cells. This activity is mediated by H_1 receptors and is of major relevance for some itch conditions such as urticaria, in which pruritus is responsive to H_1-antihistamines. Upon activation by histamine, pruritoceptors release vasodilatory neuropeptides such as substance P (SP) and calcitonin gene-related peptide (CGRP). These neuropeptides are not only released from the stimulated terminals, but also from axon collaterals which are excited by an axon reflex, thereby inducing erythema around the application site. Also, when exogenous SP is injected intradermally in high concentrations, it degranulates mast cells and consequently provokes an itch sensation.[34] However, under physiological conditions the concentrations of endogenous neuropeptides released when nociceptors are activated are too low to degranulate mast cells.[35]

Although it has been suggested that the direct excitatory effects of SP can explain itch in humans,[36] there is no experimental evidence for histamine-independent SP-induced itch in humans [37, 38] or for SP-induced excitation of nociceptors.[39] It should be noted that the amounts of SP injected intradermally, used to elicit itch in animals were unphysiologically high (2mM),[40] especially if compared to the half of the maximal concentration needed to elicit inward currents in the cell bodies of primary afferent neurons (6nM)[41] or if compared to the half maximum concentration of SP needed to produce protein extravasation in human skin (0.1 µM). Thus, reduction of scratching activity observed in SP receptor (NK_1) knock-out mice can most probably be attributed to deficits in spinal transmission mediated by NK_1 receptors at spinal neurons, or, indirectly, by presynaptic gamma-aminobutyric acid-A (GABA-A) receptors. The GABA-A receptors are inhibited by SP via NK_1 receptors[42] and, consequently, these inhibitory receptors would be more active in the NK_1 knock-outs.

There are only a few examples of mediators which can induce histamine-independent pruritus. As mentioned above, prostaglandins were found to enhance histamine-induced itch in the skin, and also to act directly as pruritogens. Neuropeptides, especially SP, have long been implicated in the mechanism of itch.[40, 43–45] There is no doubt that, at high concentrations, SP degranulates mast cells by a non-receptor mediated mechanism. However, even at high concentrations of up to 10^{-5}M, SP does not evoke any sensation or axon reflex, even though protein extravasation and vasodilation can be elicited at a concentration of 10^{-8}M without any histamine release. In contrast to rodents, physiological concentrations of endogenously released SP are obviously too low to provoke mast cell degranulation or even protein extravasation in human skin.[46] Thus, it can be concluded that SP-induced vasodilation and weal formation is mast cell independent.[47] In addition, there is probably no direct role for SP as pain or itch mediator in the periphery. This does not exclude a major role of released neuropeptides in inflammation. Trophic and immunomodulatory effects of neuropeptides have been observed at concentrations of about 10^{-11} M,[48–50] observations which might reflect their major functions under physiological conditions. In addition, in disease, the concentrations of neuropeptides in the skin might well be increased. Neuropeptides play a major role in pathophysiological mechanisms, for example in patients with chronic pain.[51]

Opioids

When directly injected intradermally opioids can activate mast cells by a non-receptor-mediated mechanism.[52] Weak opioids, like codeine, have been used as a positive control in skin prick tests. The consecutive release of histamine and mast cell tryptase can be specifically monitored by measuring tryptase concentration using dermal microdialysis following intraprobe delivery (Fig. 2.4). In contrast to morphine, the highly potent μ-opioid agonist, fentanyl, does not provoke any mast cell degranulation, even if applied at concentrations having μ-agonistic effects far exceeding those of pharmacological doses of morphine. Thus, one can conclude that morphine-induced mast cell degranulation is not mediated by μ-opioid receptors.[52] As high local concentrations of opioids are required to degranulate mast cells, systemic application of opioids in therapeutic doses does not cause pruritus by non-receptor mediated mast cell degranulation, but by central mechanisms (see also Chapter 7).

Proteinases

Although previous research has mainly focused on histamine as the main pruritic mediator in patients with itch, microdialysis has also provided evidence for mast cell-derived histamine-independent mediators, which may also induce itch. In atopic subjects, mast cell degranulation induced by compound 48/80 provokes itch, which is not suppressed by H_1-antihistamines.[53] It has been postulated that mast cell-derived tryptase is a possible candidate for this effect, as it specifically activates proteinase-activated receptors (PAR-2). Although proteinases, like papain, have been identified as histamine-independent mediators of itch decades ago,[47, 54] they received little attention until recently. However, the identification of specific proteinase-activated receptors in the membrane of afferent nerve fibres[55] has

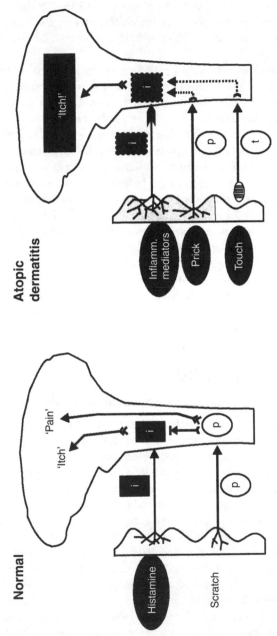

Fig. 2.4 Under physiological conditions (left panel) painful stimuli ('scratch') activates nociceptors involved in pain processing ('p'), which suppress the itch sensation at a spinal level. In atopic dermatitis (right panel) local inflammation provokes peripheral sensitization as visualized by extensive sprouting of their endings. Additionally, the spinal 'itch-neurons' ('i') are sensitized by the ongoing activity of the peripheral 'itch-neurons'. Their hyperexcitability enables normally painful ('prick') or non-painful ('touch') stimuli to generate itch. The combination of peripheral and central sensitization generates a massively enhanced itch sensation.

prompted several successful investigations of the role of PAR-2 in the *pain pathway*.[56–58] Meanwhile, there is convincing evidence for an involvement of PAR-2 in activation and sensitization of both somatic[59] and visceral afferent nerve fibres.[60–62]

Apart from its involvement in pain pathways, recent studies of PAR-2 knock-out mice indicate also a role of PAR-2 in itchy skin diseases, including atopic dermatitis.[63] Recent microdialysis data suggest that the concentration of tryptase is elevated in patients with atopic dermatitis, as would be expected from the increased numbers of tryptase-positive mast cells in this condition.[64] Activation of PAR-2 receptors may induce itch in patients with atopic dermatitis (Steinhoff M, personal communication). In this context, it is noteworthy that proteinase activity can also be found in common allergens, such as products of house dust mites. However, it is unknown whether this activity contributes only to enhanced allergic potency,[65] or whether it might also directly excite proteinase-activated receptors on sensory nerves.

The potential importance of PAR-2 signaling in the induction of dermatitis has recently been suggested by the demonstration of a marked decrease of contact dermatitis in PAR-2 knock-out mice. Because PAR-2 is expressed by various inflammatory cells, including mast cells[66] and T cells,[67] PAR-2 may be critically involved in both neurogenic and non-neurogenic inflammation of human skin.

Interaction of pain and itch

Itch modulation by pain and non-pain stimuli

It is common experience that the itch sensation can be reduced by pain caused by scratching. The inhibition of itch by painful stimuli has been shown experimentally by use of various painful thermal, mechanical and chemical stimuli. Recently, electrical stimulation via an array of pointed electrodes, a method known as cutaneous field stimulation, has also been successfully used to inhibit histamine-induced itch for several hours in an area with a diameter of up to 20 cm around a stimulated site. The large area of inhibition suggests a central mode of action.[68] Consistent with these results, itch is suppressed inside the secondary zone of capsaicin-induced mechanical hyperalgesia.[69] This central effect of nociceptor excitation by capsaicin should be clearly distinguished from the neurotoxic effect of higher concentrations of capsaicin which destroy all C-fiber terminals, including fibres that mediate itch.[70] Needless to say the latter mechanism also abolishes itching locally, until the nerve terminals have regenerated.

Not only is itch inhibited by enhanced input of pain stimuli, but also inhibition of pain processing may reduce its inhibitory effect, and thus enhance itch.[71] This phenomenon is particularly relevant to spinally administered μ-opioid receptor agonists, which are widely used in the treatment of pain and typically cause pruritus (Fig. 2.5) (see also Chapter 7).

Central inhibition of itch can also be achieved by cold stimulation.[72] In addition, histamine-induced activation of nociceptors has been shown to be temperature dependent.[73] Cooling of areas if itchy skin can reduce the activity of the primary afferents. Conversely, warming the skin would lead to an exacerbation of itch. However, as soon as the heating becomes painful, central inhibition of pruritus will counteract this effect. A summary of peripheral and central effects is given in Table 2.1.

Peripheral sensitization to pain and itch

Classical inflammatory mediators such as bradykinin, serotonin, prostanoids, and low pH have been shown to sensitize nociceptors. In addition, acute sensitization can also be achieved by inflammatory cell products, such as interleukins.[74] It has become clear that acute effects of inflammatory mediators cannot explain the prolonged changes of neuronal sensitivity observed in inflammatory processes. Regulation of gene expression induced by trophic factors, such as nerve growth factor (NGF), has been shown to play a major role in persistently increased neuronal sensitivity.[75] NGF is released in the periphery and specifically binds to TRK-A receptors located on nociceptive nerve endings. It is then conveyed via retrograde axonal transport to the dorsal root ganglion, where gene expression of neuropeptides and receptor molecules, such as the vanilloid (VR_1) receptor for capsaicin, is increased.[76] Trophic factors also initiate nerve fibre sprouting and thus change the morphology of sensory neurons. Sprouting of epidermal nerve fibres in combination with localized pain and hypersensitivity has been reported.[77, 78] It should be noted that massive crosstalk between nerve fibers and tissue cells occurs. This mutual interaction is exemplified in Figure 2.6 showing the crosstalk between nerve fibers and mast cells.

Similarly, increased intradermal nerve fibre density has been found in patients with chronic pruritus.[79, 80] Likewise, increased epidermal levels of neurotrophin 4 (NT_4) have been found in patients with atopic dermatitis[81] and massively increased serum levels of NGF and SP have been found to correlate with the severity of the disease in such patients.[82] It is known that NGF and NT_4 can sensitize nociceptors.[75, 83] Thus, the mechanisms by which peripheral nociceptors proliferate and are sensitized in patients

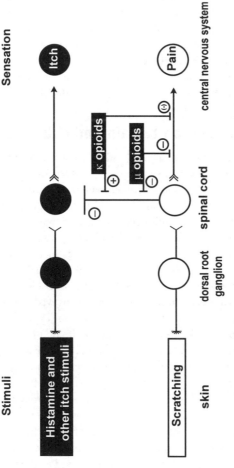

Fig. 2.5 Activation of mechanosensitive nociceptors in the skin ("scratching") can inhibit spinal "itch neurons". This pain induced inhibition can be reduced by μ-opioids. In contrast κ-agonist can increase this inhibition and thereby can act antipruritic. Modified from Andrew, D., Schmelz, M., and Ballantyne, J. C. (2003). Itch-mechanisms and mediators. In: *Progress in pain research and management.* J. O. Dostrovsky, D. B. Carr, and M. Koltzenburg (eds), Seattle: IASP Press. pp. 213–226.

Table 2.1 Peripheral and central effects on pruritus

	Effects in the skin	Spinal effects	Effect on pruritus
Temperature			
Cold	Inhibition of 'itch' units	Inhibition	Antipruritic
Warmth	Facilitation of 'itch' units	?	Pruritic
Noxious heat	Pain nociceptor activation	Inhibition	Antipruritic
μ-opioids	Histamine release	Disinhibition	Pruritic
κ-opioids	Histamine release	Inhibition	Antipruritic
Capsaicin	Neurotoxic	Inhibition	Antipruritic

with chronic itch and chronic pain are similar. However, it has not been possible to differentiate morphologically neurons that mediate itch from those that do not. There is also no evidence, at present, for a specific peripheral sensitization of itch-mediating neurons that would spare the neurons that do not mediate itch. Apart from this obvious lack of knowledge, it is very unlikely that peripheral mechanisms alone account for the obvious differences between patients with chronic itch and pain.

Central sensitization to pain and itch

There is a remarkable similarity between the phenomena associated with central sensitization to pain and itch. Activity in chemo-nociceptors leads not only to acute pain but, in addition, can sensitize second order neurons in the dorsal horn, thereby leading to increased sensitivity to pain (hyperalgesia). Two types of mechanical hyperalgesia can be differentiated. Normally painless touch sensations in the uninjured surroundings of a zone of trauma are felt as painful 'touch or brush-evoked hyperalgesia', often referred to as allodynia. Though this sensation is mediated by myelinated mechanoreceptor units, it requires ongoing activity of primary afferent C-nociceptors. A second form of mechanical hyperalgesia results in slightly painful pinprick stimulation being perceived as being more painful in the secondary zone around a focus of inflammation. This form has been called 'punctuate hyperalgesia'. The latter does not require ongoing activity of primary nociceptors. It can persist for hours following a trauma, usually much longer than touch or brush-evoked hyperalgesia.[84]

In itch processing, similar phenomena have been described: touch or brush-evoked pruritus around an itching site has been termed 'itchy skin' or alloknesis.[85–87] Like allodynia, it requires ongoing activity in primary

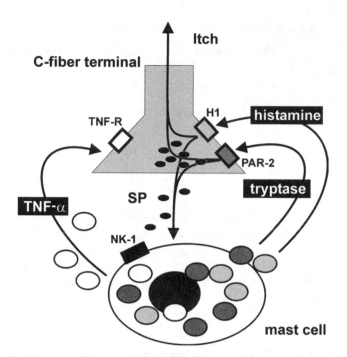

Fig. 2.6 Cross – talk between cutaneous afferent C neurone terminals and dermal mast cells. Mast cell activation releases tryptase and histamine which can activate nociceptors via PAR-2 and H1 receptors. In turn, substance P released from nociceptors can increase TNF-α, synthesis in dermal mast cells via NK1 receptors, which again can sensitize nociceptor nerve terminals. TNF = tumour necrosis factor; TNF-R = TNF receptor; H1 = histamine H1 receptor; PAR = proteinase activated receptor; NK1 = neurokinin receptor 1; SP = substance P. Modified from Yosipovitch, G., Greaves, M., and Schmelz, M. (2003). Itch. *Lancet* 361:690-694.

afferents and is elicited by low threshold mechanoreceptors (A-β fibres). Also more intense prick-induced itch sensations in the surroundings, 'hyperknesis', have been reported following histamine iontophoresis in healthy volunteers.

Although these considerations appear to be mainly of theoretical relevance, they have a great potential impact on our understanding of itch. Under the conditions of central sensitization leading to punctuate hyperknesis, normally painful stimuli are perceived as itching. This phenomenon has already been described in patients with atopy, who normally perceive painful electrical stimuli as itching.[88] Further, acetylcholine provokes itch instead of pain in patients with atopic dermatitis,[89] indicating that pain-induced inhibition of itch might be compromised in these patients. As there are a multitude of mediators and mechanisms, which are potentially algogenic in inflamed skin,[90] and thus could produce itch in a sensitized patient, a therapeutic approach, which targets single pruritic mediators, does not appear to be promising for patients with atopy. In contrast, the main therapeutic implication of this phenomenon is that a combination of centrally-acting drugs counteracting the sensitization, and topically-acting drugs counteracting the inflammation, should be more promising in ameliorating pruritus.

Although the exact mechanisms and roles of central sensitization to itch in specific, clinical conditions still have to be explored, a major role of central sensitization in patients with chronic pain is generally accepted. It should be noted that, in addition to the similarities between experimentally-induced secondary sensitization phenomena, there is emerging evidence that a corresponding interaction also exists in patients with chronic pain and chronic itch. For example, it was recently reported that, in patients with neuropathic pain, histamine iontophoresis resulted in a burning pain, rather than a pure itch sensation; pure itch would be induced by this procedure in healthy volunteers.[91] Conversely, cutaneous stimulation with an acidified solution, which provokes a purely painful sensation in normal subjects, is perceived as itching by atopic subjects, when applied in or close to their eczematous skin (Ikoma A, personal communication).

Combined peripheral and central sensitization to itch

If the consequences of central sensitization to itch are considered together with the impact of the peripheral sensitization of nociceptors described above, a coherent picture of the generation of itch emerges (Fig. 2.7). Chronic cutaneous inflammation causes local sensitization and sprouting of nociceptors in the inflamed area. In this inflammatory process, 'itch' fibres may become tonically activated, which leads to sensitization of itch processing in the spinal cord. As a consequence, normally painful stimuli can be perceived as itch. As the peripheral nociceptors are sensitized, they can be readily activated even by low intensity stimulation, and, therefore, will generate a massively enhanced input to the spinal neurons. Under normal conditions, such increased input should generate pain sensations,

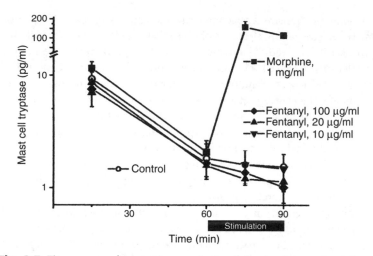

Fig. 2.7 Time course of tryptase concentration following intraprobe delivery of morphine and different concentrations of fentanyl (black bar) by dermal microdialysis. Note, that only morphine provokes mast cell tryptase release. Data are means ± SEM ($n = 7$).

which in turn would suppress itch. However, when itch processing is sensitized, subjects will perceive intense pruritus instead. Both phenomena can co-exist, but on different time scales. Thus, although scratching may inhibit itch, it may also be perceived as itch by a centrally sensitized patient. This latter phenomenon may promote a vicious itch-scratch cycle.

Conclusions

• The mechanisms of peripheral sensitization of C-fibres to pain and pruritus are similar, some mechanisms may be even identical.
• Why inflammatory processes usually cause pain, and only sometimes cause itch is not known.
• Probably not all clinically relevant mediators of pruritus are known.

Acknowledgments

This work was supported by the Deutsche Forschungsgemeinschaft (SFB 353).

References

1. von Frey M. (1922). Zur Physiologie der Juckempfindung. *Arch Neerl Physiol* 7:142–5.

2. Torebjörk HE, Ochoa P. (1981). Pain and itch from Fiber stimulation. *Soc Neurosci Abstr* 7:228.

3. Schmelz M, Schmidt R, Bickel A, Handwerker HO, Torebjörk HE. (1997). Specific C–receptors for itch in human skin. *J Neurosci* 17:8003–8.

4. Handwerker HO, Forster C, Kirchhoff C. (1991). Discharge patterns of human C-fibers induced by itching and burning stimuli. *J Neurophysiol* 66:307–15.

5. Perl ER. (1996). Cutaneous polymodal receptors: characteristics and plasticity. *Prog Brain Res* 113:21–37.

6. Wahlgren CF, Ekblom A. (1996). Two-point discrimination of itch in patients with atopic dermatitis and healthy subjects. *Acta Derm Venereol* 76:48–51.

7. Schmidt R, Schmelz M, Ringkamp M, Handwerker HO, Torebjörk HE. (1997). Innervation territories of mechanically activated C nociceptor units in human skin. *J Neurophysiol* 78:2641–8.

8. Meyer RA, Campbell JN. (1988). A novel electrophysiological technique for locating cutaneous nociceptive and chemospecific receptors. *Brain Res* 441:81–6.

9. Lynn B. (1991). 'Silent' nociceptors in the skin. *Trends Neurosci* 14:95.

10. Meyer RA, Davis KD, Cohen RH, Treede RD, Campbell JN. (1991). Mechanically insensitive afferents (MIAs) in cutaneous nerves of monkey. *Brain Res* 561:252–61.

11. Lynn B. (1992). Capsaicin: actions on C fibre afferents that may be involved in itch. *Skin Pharmacol* 5:9–13.

12. Schmidt RF, Schaible HG, Messlinger K, Hanesch U, Pawlak M. (1994). Silent and active nociceptors: structure, functions and clinical implications. GF Gebhart, DL Hammind, and TS Jensen (eds), Seattle: IASP Press. pp. 213–50.

13. Schmelz M, Schmid R, Handwerker HO, Torebjörk HE. (2000). Encoding of burning pain from capsaicin-treated human skin in two categories of unmyelinated nerve fibres. *Brain* 123 Pt 3:560–71.

14. Yosipovitch G. (2002). Proceedings of the 1st International Workshop for the Study of Itch.

15. Hägermark O, Strandberg K. (1977). Pruritogenic activity of prostaglandin E2. *Acta Derm Venereol* 57:37–43.

16. Hägermark O, Strandberg K, Hamberg M. (1977). Potentiation of itch and flare responses in human skin by prostaglandins E2 and H2 and a prostaglandin endoperoxide analog. *J Invest Dermatol* 69:527–30.

17. Woodward DF, Nieves AL, Hawley SB, Joseph R, Merlino GF, Spada CS. (1995). The pruritogenic and inflammatory effects of prostanoids in the conjunctiva. *J Ocul Pharmacol Ther* 11:339–47.

18. Neisius U, Olsson R, Rukwied R, Lischetzki G, Schmelz M. (2002). Prostaglandin E2 induces vasodilation and pruritus, but no protein extravasation in atopic dermatitis and controls. *J Am Acad Dermatol* **47**:28–32.

19. Hägermark O. (1992). Peripheral and central mediators of itch. *Skin Pharmacol* **5**:1–8.

20. Weisshaar E, Ziethen B, Rohl FW, Gollnick H. (1999). The antipruritic effect of a 5-HT$_3$ receptor antagonist (tropisetron) is dependent on mast cell depletion—an experimental study. *Exp Dermatol* **8**:254–60.

21. Vogelsang M, Heyer G, Hornstein OP. (1995). Acetylcholine induces different cutaneous sensations in atopic and non- atopic subjects. *Acta Derm Venereol* **75**:434–6.

22. Juhlin L, Michaelsson G. (1969). Cutaneous vascular reactions to prostaglandins in healthy subjects and in patients with urticaria and atopic dermatitis. *Acta Derm Venereol* **49**:251–61.

23. Kingston WP, Greaves MW. (1985). Actions of prostaglandin E2 metabolites on skin microcirculation. *Agents Actions* **16**:13–4.

24. Sabroe RA, Kennedy CT, Archer CB. (1997). The effects of topical doxepin on responses to histamine, substance P and prostaglandin E2 in human skin. *Br J Dermatol* **137**:386–90.

25. Sciberras DG, Goldenberg MM, Bolognese JA, James I, Baber NS. (1987). Inflammatory responses to intradermal injection of platelet activating factor, histamine and prostaglandin E2 in healthy volunteers: a double blind investigation. *Br J Clin Pharmacol* **24**:753–61.

26. Lischetzki G, Rukwied R, Handwerker HO, Schmelz M. (2001). Nociceptor activation and protein extravasation induced by inflammatory mediators in human skin. *Eur J Pain* **5**:49–57.

27. McMahon SB, Koltzenburg M. (1992). Itching for an explanation. *Trends Neurosci* **15**:497–501.

28. Andrew D, Craig AD. (2001). Spinothalamic lamina I neurons selectively sensitive to histamine: a central neural pathway for itch. *Nat Neurosci* **4**:72–7.

29. Craig AD. (2002). How do you feel? Interoception: the sense of the physiological condition of the body. *Nat Rev Neurosci* **3**:655–66.

30. Hsieh JC, Hägermark O, Stahle-Backdahl M, Ericson K, Eriksson L, Stone-Elander S, Ingvar M. (1994). Urge to scratch represented in the human cerebral cortex during itch. *J Neurophysiol* **72**:3004–8.

31. Darsow U, Drzezga A, Frisch M, Munz F, Weilke F, Bartenstein P, Schwaiger M, Ring J. (2000). Processing of histamine-induced itch in the human cerebral cortex: a correlation analysis with dermal reactions. *J Invest Dermatol* **115**:1029–33.

32. Drzezga A, Darsow U, Treede RD, Siebner H, Frisch M, Munz F, Weilke F, Ring J, Schwaiger M, Bartenstein P. (2001). Central activation by histamine-induced itch: analogies to pain processing: a correlational analysis of O-15 H2O positron emission tomography studies. *Pain* **92**:295–305.

33. Magerl W, Westerman RA, Mohner B, Handwerker HO. (1990). Properties of transdermal histamine iontophoresis: differential effects of season, gender, and body region. *J Invest Dermatol* **94**:347–52.

34. Hägermark O, Hokfelt T, Pernow B. (1978). Flare and itch induced by substance P in human skin. *J Invest Dermatol* **71**:233–5.

35. Schmelz M, Zeck S, Raithel M, Rukwied R. (1999). Mast cell tryptase in dermal neurogenic inflammation. *Clin Exp Allergy* **29**:695–702.

36. Wallengren J, Hakanson R. (1987). Effects of substance P, neurokinin A and calcitonin gene-related peptide in human skin and their involvement in sensory nerve-mediated responses. *Eur J Pharmacol* **143**:267–73.

37. Weidner C, Klede M, Rukwied R, Lischetzki G, Neisius U, Skov PS, Petersen LJ, Schmelz M. (2000). Acute effects of substance P and calcitonin gene-related peptide in human skin—a microdialysis study. *J Invest Dermatol* **115**:1015–20.

38. Schmelz M, Petersen LJ. (2001). Neurogenic inflammation in human and rodent skin. *News Physiol Sci* **16**:33–7.

39. Kessler W, Kirchhoff C, Reeh PW, Handwerker HO. (1992). Excitation of cutaneous afferent nerve endings in vitro by a combination of inflammatory mediators and conditioning effect of substance P. *Exp Brain Res* **91**:467–76.

40. Andoh T, Nagasawa T, Satoh M, Kuraishi Y. (1998). Substance P induction of itch-associated response mediated by cutaneous NK1 tachykinin receptors in mice. *J Pharmacol Exp Ther* **286**:1140–5.

41. Akasu T, Ishimatsu M, Yamada K. (1996). Tachykinins cause inward current through NK1 receptors in bullfrog sensory neurons. *Brain Res* **713**:160–7.

42. Yamada K, Akasu T. (1996). Substance P suppresses GABA-A receptor function via protein kinase C in primary sensory neurones of bullfrogs. *J Physiol* **496(Pt 2)**:439–49.

43. Heyer G, Hornstein OP, Handwerker HO. (1991). Reactions to intradermally injected substance P and topically applied mustard oil in atopic dermatitis patients. *Acta Derm Venereol* **71**:291–5.

44. Wallengren J, Akesson A, Scheja A, Sundler F. (1996). Occurrence and distribution of peptidergic nerve fibers in skin biopsies from patients with systemic sclerosis. *Acta Derm Venereol* **76**:126–8.

45. Giannetti A, Girolomoni G. (1989). Skin reactivity to neuropeptides in atopic dermatitis. *Br J Dermatol* **121**:681–8.

46. Sauerstein K, Klede M, Hilliges M, Schmelz M. (2000). Electrically evoked neuropeptide release and neurogenic inflammation differ between rat and human skin. *J Physiol* **529(Pt 3)**:803–10.

47. Rajka G. (1969). Latency and duration of pruritus elicited by trypsin in aged patients with itching eczema and psoriasis. *Acta Derm Venereol* **49**:401–3.

48. Noveral JP, Grunstein MM. (1995). Tachykinin regulation of airway smooth muscle cell proliferation. *Am J Physiol* **269**:L339–43.

49. Parenti A, Amerini S, Ledda F, Maggi CA, Ziche M. (1996). The tachykinin NK1 receptor mediates the migration-promoting effect of substance P on human skin fibroblasts in culture. *Naunyn Schmiedebergs Arch Pharmacol* **353**:475–81.

50. Lambert RW, Granstein RD. (1998). Neuropeptides and Langerhans cells. *Exp Dermatol* **7**:73–80.

51. Weber M, Birklein F, Neundorfer B, Schmelz M. (2001). Facilitated neurogenic inflammation in complex regional pain syndrome. *Pain* **91**:251–7.

52. Church MK, Clough GF. (1999). Human skin mast cells: in vitro and in vivo studies. *Ann Allergy Asthma Immunol* **83**:471–5.

53. Rukwied R, Lischetzki G, McGlone F, Heyer G, Schmelz M. (2000). Mast cell mediators other than histamine induce pruritus in atopic dermatitis patients: a dermal microdialysis study. *Br J Dermatol* **142**:1114–20.

54. Hägermark O. (1973). Influence of antihistamines, sedatives, and aspirin on experimental itch. *Acta Derm Venereol* **53**:363–8.

55. Steinhoff M, Vergnolle N, Young SH, Tognetto M, Amadesi S, Ennes HS, Trevisani M, Hollenberg MD, Wallace JL, Caughey GH, Mitchell SE, Williams LM, Geppetti P, Mayer EA, Bunnett NW. (2000). Agonists of proteinase-activated receptor 2 induce inflammation by a neurogenic mechanism. *Nat Med* **6**:151–8.

56. Vergnolle N, Bunnett NW, Sharkey KA, Brussee V, Compton SJ, Grady EF, Cirino G, Gerard N, Basbaum AI, Andrade-Gordon P, Hollenberg MD, Wallace JL. (2001). Proteinase-activated receptor-2 and hyperalgesia: A novel pain pathway. *Nat Med* **7**:821–6.

57. Vergnolle N, Wallace JL, Bunnett NW, Hollenberg MD. (2001). Protease-activated receptors in inflammation, neuronal signaling and pain. *Trends Pharmacol Sci* **22**:146–52.

58. Fiorucci S, Distrutti E. (2002). Role of PAR2 in pain and inflammation. *Trends Pharmacol Sci* **23**:153–5.

59. Kawabata A, Kawao N, Kuroda R, Tanaka A, Itoh H, Nishikawa H. (2001). Peripheral PAR-2 triggers thermal hyperalgesia and nociceptive responses in rats. *Neuroreport* **12**:715–9.

60. Corvera CU, Dery O, McConalogue K, Gamp P, Thoma M, Al-Ani B, Caughey GH, Hollenberg MD, Bunnett NW. (1999). Thrombin and mast cell tryptase regulate guinea-pig myenteric neurons through proteinase-activated receptors-1 and -2. *J Physiol* **517**(Pt 3):741–56.

61. Hoogerwerf WA, Zou L, Shenoy M, Sun D, Micci MA, Lee-Hellmich H, Xiao SY, Winston JH, Pasricha PJ. (2001). The proteinase-activated receptor 2 is involved in nociception. *J Neurosci* **21**:9036–42.

62. Coelho AM, Vergnolle N, Guiard B, Fioramonti J, Bueno L. (2002). Proteinases and proteinase-activated receptor 2: a possible role to promote visceral hyperalgesia in rats. *Gastroenterology* **122**:1035–47.

63. Kawagoe J, Takizawa T, Matsumoto J, Tamiya M, Meek SE, Smith AJ, Hunter GD, Plevin R, Saito N, Kanke T, Fujii M, Wada Y. (2002). Effect of protease-activated receptor-2 deficiency on allergic dermatitis in the mouse ear. *Jpn J Pharmacol* **88**:77–84.

64. Jarvikallio A, Naukkarinen A, Harvima IT, Aalto ML, Horsmanheimo M. (1997). Quantitative analysis of tryptase- and chymase-containing mast cells in atopic dermatitis and nummular eczema. *Br J Dermatol* **136**:871–7.

65. Gough L, Schulz O, Sewell HF, Shakib F. (1999). The cysteine protease activity of the major dust mite allergen Der p 1 selectively enhances the immunoglobulin E antibody response. *J Exp Med* **190**:1897–902.

66. D'Andrea MR, Rogahn CJ, Andrade-Gordon P. (2000). Localization of protease-activated receptors-1 and -2 in human mast cells: indications for an amplified mast cell degranulation cascade. *Biotech Histochem* **75**:85–90.

67. Bar-Shavit R, Maoz M, Yongjun Y, Groysman M, Dekel I, Katzav S. (2002). Signalling pathways induced by protease-activated receptors and integrins in T cells. *Immunology* **105**:35–46.

68. Nilsson HJ, Levinsson A, Schouenborg J. (1997). Cutaneous field stimulation (CFS): a new powerful method to combat itch. *Pain* **71**:49–55.

69. Brull SJ, Atanassoff PG, Silverman DG, Zhang J, Lamotte RH. (1999). Attenuation of experimental pruritus and mechanically evoked dysesthesiae in an area of cutaneous allodynia. *Somatosens Mot Res* **16**:299–303.

70. Simone DA, Nolano M, Johnson T, Wendelschafer-Crabb G, Kennedy WR. (1998). Intradermal injection of capsaicin in humans produces degeneration and subsequent reinnervation of epidermal nerve fibers: correlation with sensory function. *J Neurosci* **18**:8947–59.

71. Atanassoff PG, Brull SJ, Zhang J, Greenquist K, Silverman DG, Lamotte RH. (1999). Enhancement of experimental pruritus and mechanically evoked dysesthesiae with local anesthesia. *Somatosens Mot Res* **16**:291–8.

72. Bromm B, Scharein E, Darsow U, Ring J. (1995). Effects of menthol and cold on histamine-induced itch and skin reactions in man. *Neurosci Lett* **187**:157–60.

73. Mizumura K, Koda H. (1999). Potentiation and suppression of the histamine response by raising and lowering the temperature in canine visceral polymodal receptors in vitro. *Neurosci Lett* **266**:9–12.

74. Kidd BL, Urban LA. (2001). Mechanisms of inflammatory pain. *Br J Anaesth* **87**:3–11.

75. Shu XQ, Llinas A, Mendell LM. (1999). Effects of trkB and trkC neurotrophin receptor agonists on thermal nociception: a behavioral and electrophysiological study. *Pain* **80**:463–70.

76. Bennett DL. (2001). Neurotrophic factors: important regulators of nociceptive function. *Neuroscientist* **7**:13–7.

77. Bohm-Starke N, Hilliges M, Falconer C, Rylander E. (1998). Increased intraepithelial innervation in women with vulvar vestibulitis syndrome. *Gynecol Obstet Invest* **46**:256–60.

78. Bohm-Starke N, Hilliges M, Brodda-Jansen G, Rylander E, Torebjörk E. (2001). Psychophysical evidence of nociceptor sensitization in vulvar vestibulitis syndrome. *Pain* **94**:177–83.

79. Sugiura H, Omoto M, Hirota Y, Danno K, Uehara M. (1997). Density and fine structure of peripheral nerves in various skin lesions of atopic dermatitis. *Arch Dermatol Res* **289**:125–31.

80. Urashima R, Mihara M. (1998). Cutaneous nerves in atopic dermatitis. A histological, immunohistochemical and electron microscopic study. *Virchows Arch* **432**:363–70.

81. Grewe M, Vogelsang K, Ruzicka T, Stege H, Krutmann J. (2000). Neurotrophin-4 production by human epidermal keratinocytes: increased expression in atopic dermatitis. *J Invest Dermatol* **114**:1108–12.

82. Toyoda M, Nakamura M, Makino T, Hino T, Kagoura M, Morohashi M. (2002). Nerve growth factor and substance P are useful plasma markers of disease activity in atopic dermatitis. *Br J Dermatol* **147**:71–9.

83. Romero MI, Rangappa N, Li L, Lightfoot E, Garry MG, Smith GM. (2000). Extensive sprouting of sensory afferents and hyperalgesia induced by conditional expression of nerve growth factor in the adult spinal cord. *J Neurosci* **20**:4435–45.

84. LaMotte RH. (1986). James Daniel Hardy (1904–1985). Tribute to a pioneer in pain psychophysics. *Pain* **27**:127–30.

85. Bickford RGL. 1938. Experiments relating to itch sensation, its peripheral mechanism and central pathways. *Clin Sci* **3**:377–86.

86. Simone DA, Alreja M, LaMotte RH. (1991). Psychophysical studies of the itch sensation and itchy skin ("alloknesis") produced by intracutaneous injection of histamine. *Somatosens Mot Res* **8**:271–9.

87. Heyer G, Ulmer FJ, Schmitz J, Handwerker HO. (1995). Histamine-induced itch and alloknesis (itchy skin) in atopic eczema patients and controls. *Acta Derm Venereol* **75**:348–52.

88. Nilsson HJ, Schouenborg J. (1999). Differential inhibitory effect on human nociceptive skin senses induced by local stimulation of thin cutaneous fibers. *Pain* **80**:103–12 .

89. Groene D, Martus P, Heyer G. (2001). Doxepin affects acetylcholine induced cutaneous reactions in atopic eczema. *Exp Dermatol* **10**:110–7.

90. Reeh PW, Kress M. (1995). Effects of Classical Algogens. *Semin Neurosci* **7**:221–6.

91. Baron R, Schwarz K, Kleinert A, Schattschneider J, Wasner G. (2001). Histamine-induced itch converts into pain in neuropathic hyperalgesia. *Neuroreport* **12**:3475–8.

3

Clinical assessment of patients with pruritus

Zbigniew Zylicz

The clinical context of pruritus

Pruritus is not a disease—it is a symptom that may accompany many conditions. In advanced diseases, it is rarely the sole expression of the underlying disorder. Thus, when evaluating patients with pruritus, it is necessary to assess the pruritus in the context of the patient's total physical and psychological condition.

Interestingly, some patients with severe pruritus in disseminated malignant disease experience little or no pain.[1] Others with severe pain experience pruritus only when their pain is controlled (see Chapter 2). Some patients experience pain and pruritus simultaneously.[2] A few patients experience pruritus as an adverse effect of opioid analgesics. So it is important that a thorough history is obtained of all symptoms and of their temporal relationship to pruritus, as well as details of all medication being taken.

Symptoms that may accompany pruritus

Enquire not only about the pruritus and pain,[3] but also about fatigue,[4] constipation,[5] and nausea and vomiting. These symptoms may be associated with the increased endogenous opioidergic tone that is increasingly associated with pruritus.[4] One symptom that is less frequently related to increased opioidergic tone is cough. Chatila, Bergasa, *et al.* reported one case of pruritus due to benign recurrent intrahepatic cholestasis that was accompanied by intractable dry cough.[6] This type of cough, which does not respond to codeine, may be evoked by increased opioidergic tone, for example, after rapid injection of fentanyl.[7–11] What has this type of cough in common with pruritus?

Pain, pruritus, cough, and probably many other signals from the periphery are modulated by central inhibitory mechanisms. This has been shown most clearly for pain.[12] Increased opioidergic tone is responsible for an increase in pain threshold. However, the same increased opioidergic tone causes a decrease in pruritus threshold.[13, 14] The serotoninergic, adrenergic, and GABAergic systems are also involved in central inhibition, although the responses from these systems are more complicated.

In the past we have reported on a series of patients with pruritus, who responded to administration of paroxetine (reference 15 and Zylicz Z, Krajnik M, van Sorge AA, Costantini M. (2003). Paroxetine in the treatment of severe non-dermatological pruritus: a randomized, controlled trial. *J Pain Symptom Manage* (in press)). Later we described five patients with persistent distressing cough who responded to paroxetine (Zylicz Z, Krajnik M. (2003). What has dry cough in common with pruritus? Treatment of dry cough with paroxetine. *J Pain Symptom Manage* (in press)). Two of the patients also simultaneously experienced severe pruritus, and both symptoms were controlled by paroxetine. It is hypothesized that both symptoms may result from decreased central inhibition, which may be restored by serotonin reuptake inhibitors (SSRI).

In all our patients, cough responded to paroxetine. The effect was rapid and prolonged. In two patients, where it was possible to observe, the onset of antitussive effect was within 20–30 minutes after drug administration. Paroxetine was not inhibiting productive cough allowing patients to expectorate. After discontinuing codeine in all patients, expectorating was increased. Interestingly, all the patients were women. This could be coincidental but women are known to have a lower threshold for dry cough.[16–18]

Curiously, nausea after taking paroxetine was not seen in patients with cough alone. According to our previous observations during a controlled trial, nausea was nearly obligatory for the patients with pruritus responding to paroxetine (Zylicz Z, Krajnik M, van Sorge AA, Costantini M. (2003). Paroxetine in the treatment of severe non-dermatological pruritus: a randomized, controlled trial. *J Pain Symptom Manage* (in press)). Patients with pruritus responded to paroxetine usually after 2–3 days, while patients with cough in the present series responded usually within hours. This suggests that cough and pruritus are two different phenomena and are responding to SSRIs differently. It is tempting to speculate, that in cough 5-HT_1 and particularly 5-HT_{1A} receptors are involved, while in pruritus 5-HT_2 and 5-HT_3 may be important. The latter receptors may also be responsible for transient emetogenesis.

Psychological disorders such as neurosis or depression may also accompany pruritus (see Chapter 11). Thus, pruritus should be always seen in context of the whole patient and his or her suffering.

Temporal relationships

When there is an associated skin rash, it is important to establish whether the rash appeared first, before the pruritus, or vice versa, particularly because the rash is sometimes the result of scratching or rubbing. Intensive and long-standing rubbing may be the reason of secondary inflammation and focal accumulation of amyloid, which in its turn may perpetuate pruritus.[19] Acute localized pruritus of only several days' duration is less suggestive of underlying systemic disease than chronic progressive generalized pruritus.

Age of onset

The frequency of pruritus increases with age.[20] However, the prevalence of allergy accompanied by pruritus, for example, atopic dermatitis, is highest in children. Many old people suffer from 'senile pruritus'. This often gets worse in the winter ('winter itch'), and is exacerbated by xerosis and psychological distress.[21] Xerosis alone cannot explain the whole phenomenon,[22] notably its response to immunosuppressive drugs.[23, 24] It has been suggested that senile pruritus may be related to nerve injury in ageing skin and could be thought of as the equivalent of phantom pain.[25] Indeed, loss of neurons in ageing skin is probably responsible for impaired thermal regulation, reduced tactile sensitivity, and impaired pain perception.[26] Loss of neurons in the skin could also be responsible for pruritus as a result of reduced neural inhibition.

Is the pruritus associated with skin disease?

In the evaluation it is important to determine whether the pruritus is related to primary skin disease or to a systemic disease accompanied by a skin disorder and pruritus. Pruritus is a frequent symptom of skin disease. In patients with inflammatory skin disease, the pruritus is generally assumed to be a response to one or more chemical mediators, including histamine, neuropeptides, and eicosanoids. However, there are some dermatoses that may be difficult to recognize but severely pruritic, including atopic dermatitis, bullous pemphigoid, contact dermatitis, dermatitis herpetiformis, fibreglass dermatitis, miliaria, pediculosis, scabies, urticaria, and xerosis. Therefore, patients presenting solely with pruritus should first be examined by a dermatologist to exclude these dermatoses, especially because they are readily treatable.

Asking about any recent visits to tropical countries may help to diagnose an unusual parasitic or fungal infection and is good clinical practice. In some patients, pruritus may persist even when the skin disease is in remission. This may be due to central sensitization (see Chapter 2). However, in most cases, skin diseases are well defined and easily recognizable.

Contact dermatitis should be thought of if the pruritus is localized. For example, contact with wool may cause allergy and pruritus. Pruritus may also be caused by latex and chromium used in leather tanning.[27] In this situation, the pruritus may be limited to the feet or the belt area.

Occasionally, skin biopsy may be necessary in order to determine the cause. Reviewing old medical records may also help with diagnosis. A history of severe pruritus in childhood due to atopic dermatitis may explain why an elderly patient develops pruritus in conjunction with a disorder that is not typically associated with it. Surgical scars may be highly pruritic in patients with a past history of severe pruritus.

Is the pruritus localized or generalized?

Localized pruritus usually is not a consequence of systemic disease. Fixed localized itching may be due to organic neurological disease, for example, in segmental neurofibromatosis or in notalgia paraesthetica. Sometimes neuropathic pruritus begins in one area but later affects the whole body as a result of central sensitization.

Some forms of pruritus are by definition local, for example, conjunctival,[28] vaginal (associated with infection),[29] or anal (venous congestion of the perianal skin).[30] On the other hand, occasionally, perianal pruritus may be a symptom of prostate cancer, and pruritus vulvae a symptom of cervical cancer (see Chapter 8).

Generalized pruritus may initially be localized. Although in many systemic diseases pruritus may be generalized, some areas of the body may be more severely affected than others. Ask and look for the specific 'itch points'. These are specific places on the skin that, if stroked, induce pruritus in a much wider area, not always in a dermatomal distribution.

Is the pruritus related to treatment?

Review the present and past drug medication thoroughly. Many drugs can induce pruritus through an allergic reaction, often acute urticaria.

Sometimes acute urticaria is delayed several days and may occur after discontinuation of a drug. This happens, for example, after a course of amoxicillin. Other drugs, for example, chloroquine, may cause pruritus without a rash (Table 3.1). Impaired metabolism of this drug in patients without certain liver enzymes causes accumulation of metabolites that may be responsible for the pruritus.[31] Rarely, anal pruritus may be caused by anticancer drugs (see Chapter 8).[32]

Table 3.1 Drugs and treatment methods occasionally inducing pruritus without rash (alphabetically)

allopurinol	insulin
amiodarone	isotretinoin and other retinoids
amitriptylline	ketoconazole
ampicillin	metronidazole
aspirin	miconazole
atenolol	morphine
bleomycin	niacin
butorphanol	NSAIDs
captopril	oestrogens
cephalosporins	oral contraceptives
clonidine	phenolphthalein
colchicine	polimyxin B
colistin	photochemotherapy (PUVA)
coumarins	probenecid
dexamethazone	progesterones
diazoxide	propylthiouracil
dobutamine	quinidine
enalapril	starch, hydroxyethylstarch
fentanyl	sulfonamides
furosemide	sulfonylureas
gold	suramin
heparins	warfarin
hydrochlorothiazide	vitamin B complex
imipramine	

Morphine and other opioids also induce pruritus without a rash.[33] Rapid intravenous injection of high doses of dexamethazone can induce vulval pruritus without a rash.[34] The reason for this is unknown.

Heavy metals such as lead, mercury, platinum, and gold, used for therapy of various systemic disorders, may be highly neurotoxic and can cause pruritus.[35–45] Pruritus due to heavy metals may be localized or generalized. Heavy metals used in dentistry can cause generalized pruritus.[46] Finally, natural remedies may induce difficult-to-diagnose pruritus, mainly because our knowledge about them is limited.

When to suspect systemic disease

Among all patients seeking medical attention for pruritus, the prevalence of underlying systemic disease has been reported to be 10–50%.[47–49] When itching is a manifestation of systemic disease, the cause may be also evident in the skin itself, as dry skin in hyperparathyroidism, warm and moist skin in thyrotoxicosis, or cutaneous candidiasis in diabetes mellitus. However, more often, systemic disease causes itching in healthy-looking skin.[50] Pruritus that is migratory in timing and distribution may be secondary to internal malignancy. Sometimes pruritus is a prodrome of systemic disease and may be experienced by patients for years before the malignancy is diagnosed. This is especially true for non-Hodgkin's lymphoma and polycythaemia vera (see Chapter 10).

Factors that precipitate pruritus

Ingestion of certain kinds of food, for example, pepper, nuts, red wine, and chocolate, may precipitate pruritus. Interestingly, this kind of pruritus may not be related to true allergy, as the skin allergy tests to these substances remain negative. Also H_1-antihistamines do not relieve or prevent this kind of pruritus. It is thus probable that substances derived from these food products may provoke release of the substance P from the nerve endings and hence induce pruritus (see Chapter 2). A similar mechanism is suspected in migraine precipitated by alcohol and certain foods.[51] Elimination of the causal food from the diet is successful in the treatment of this kind of pruritus.

Exercise may also be responsible for cholinergic stimulation and cause massive histamine release, extensive pruritus, and even anaphylaxis.[52–56] Stress may precipitate pruritus through adrenergic stimulation.[57] Water, especially showers, is responsible for aquagenic pruritus,[58] which may be a symptom of polycythaemia vera or be an isolated symptom in a healthy person (see Chapter 10).[59, 60]

Factors that relieve pruritus

Scratching may relieve pruritus, mainly by causing pain. Distraction can also alleviate pruritus. Some drugs administered for other reasons, may unexpectedly relieve pruritus, for example, antidepressants.[61] In the case of some of them, the antipruritic activity is probably related to strong anti-histamine activity. Other antidepressants, like paroxetine, probably allevi-ate pruritus by restoring the central inhibition processes (reference 15 and Zylicz Z, Krajnik M. (2003). What has dry cough in common with pruritus? Treatment of dry cough with paroxetine. *J Pain Symptom Manage* (in press)).

One patient with severe pruritus caused by primary biliary cirrhosis told us that the only day in the last decades she could recall without pruritus was the day after a gynaecological operation. Morphine or another opioid was probably given as postoperative analgesia. She was treated with oral codeine and her pruritus remained under control for many years.[62]

Changes in the climate can have a major effect on pruritus. A warm dry climate may diminish itching in polycythaemia vera, whereas too much sun may increase itching due to sun dermatosis.[20] The wet cold winters in Northern Europe cause many old people suffering from pruritus to spend time in Spain, Italy, or Greece.

Physical examination

A thorough physical examination, including palpation of lymph nodes, liver, and spleen as well as pelvic and rectal examinations, is important. Skin examination should involve assessment of its colour (e.g. iron deficiency anaemia, jaundice), moisture (e.g. xerosis), scaling (e.g. pityriasis), infections (e.g. candidiasis), and infestations (e.g. scabies). Analysis of secondary effects of scratching may give some information about the severity of pruritus. Right-handed people will scratch their left back more intensively. Neurological examination, especially testing of sensitivity, may disclose abnormalities associated with peripheral neuropathy or central involvement.

Laboratory investigations

Evaluation of the pruritic patient without skin manifestations should be directed at determining systemic causes. If the index of suspicion for

> ## Box 3.1 Laboratory tests in generalized pruritus
>
> - Complete blood count including differential white cell count
> - Liver enzymes, bilirubin, albumin
> - Plasma uric acid and renal function tests
> - Thyroid function tests
> - Faeces for occult blood and parasite eggs
> - Plasma and urine glucose
> - HIV antibody (if risk factors are present)
> - Full urine examination including urine microscopy
> - Chest radiograph

systemic disease is low based on the history, review of systems, and physical examination, a 2-week trial of symptomatic therapy can be prescribed before considering laboratory tests (Box 3.1).

When to suspect a psychogenic origin of pruritus

Is pruritus present during night? Most of organic pruritic conditions tend to get worse at night and cause sleeplessness and fatigue. However, in many psychogenic conditions complicated by pruritus, patients obtain relief when sleeping (see Chapter 11). Itching described by patient as insects crawling over the skin is often psychoneurotic in origin (only if skin infestation by insects is excluded!). Most patients are especially uncomfortable in bed, because of warmth and little to distract their attention.

The role of depression, stress, and anxiety in causing pruritus is unknown. It may be difficult to differentiate primary from secondary psychiatric illness, because depression and anxiety are common consequences of chronic itching. Pruritus of unknown cause may be due to a psychologically reduced threshold to pruritogenic stimuli.[63] Patients need psychological support and some of them may require mild anxiolytics, antidepressants, or psychiatric consultation. As said before, antidepressants probably restore central inhibition of pruritus (Zylicz Z, Krajnik M. (2003). What has dry cough in common with pruritus? Treatment of dry cough with paroxetine. *J Pain Symptom Manage* (in press)), which may be decreased in the presence of increased opioidergic tone.

Pruritus of unknown origin

Despite a carefully taken history, review of systems, physical examination, and laboratory tests, no cause can be established in some patients.[60, 63, 64] Such patients should be followed up regularly because pruritus is occasionally the prodrome of a disease that will emerge at a later date.

Conclusions

- When evaluating patients with pruritus, it is necessary to assess the pruritus in the context of the patient's total physical and psychological condition.
- Pain (or lack of it, despite obvious pathology), fatigue, nausea and vomiting, constipation, and cough may be associated with pruritus.
- The above symptoms may result from increased opioidergic tone and decreased central inhibition of other than pain processes.
- Patients presenting solely with pruritus should first be examined by a dermatologist to exclude skin diseases.
- Localized pruritus usually is rarely if ever a consequence of systemic disease.
- Many drugs may cause pruritus without a rash.
- The prevalence of systemic disease among the patients with severe, generalized pruritus has been reported to be 10–50%.
- Patients with pruritus should be followed up regularly because pruritus is occasionally the prodrome of a disease that will emerge at a later date.

References

1. Zylicz Z, Krajnik M. (1999). Pruritus in cancer. Rare, but sometimes worse than pain [in Dutch]. *Ned Tijdschr Geneeskd* **143**:1937–40.
2. Twycross RG. (1981). Pruritus and pain in en cuirass breast cancer. *Lancet* **2**:696.
3. Teofoli P, Procacci P, Maresca M, Lotti T. (1996). Itch and pain. *Int J Dermatol* **35**:159–66.
4. Jones EA, Bergasa NV. (1999). The pathogenesis and treatment of pruritus and fatigue in patients with PBC. *Eur J Gastroenterol Hepatol* **11**:623–31.
5. Schuster MM. (1977). Constipation and anorectal disorders. *Clin Gastroenterol* **6**:643–58.

6. Chatila R, Bergasa NV, Lagarde S, West AB. (1996). Intractable cough and abnormal pulmonary function in benign recurrent intrahepatic cholestasis. *Am J Gastroenterol* **91**:2215–19.

7. Tsou CH, Luk HN, Chiang SC, Hsin ST, Wang JH. (2002). Fentanyl-induced coughing and airway hyperresponsiveness. *Acta Anaesthesiol Sin* **40**:165–72.

8. Tweed WA, Dakin D. (2001). Explosive coughing after bolus fentanyl injection. *Anesth Analg* **92**:1442–3.

9. Gin T, Chui PT. (1992). Coughing after fentanyl. *Can J Anaesth* **39**:406.

10. Phua WT, Teh BT, Jong W, Lee TL, Tweed WA. (1991). Tussive effect of a fentanyl bolus. *Can J Anaesth* **38**:330–4.

11. Ananthanarayan C. (1990). Tussive effect of fentanyl. *Anaesthesia* **45**:595.

12. Kakigi R. (1994). Diffuse noxious inhibitory control. Reappraisal by pain-related somatosensory evoked potentials following CO_2 laser stimulation. *J Neurol Sci* **125**:198–205.

13. Jones EA, Dekker LR. (2000). Florid opioid withdrawal-like reaction precipitated by naltrexone in a patient with chronic cholestasis. *Gastroenterology* **118**:431–2.

14. Jones EA, Bergasa NV. (1999). The pruritus of cholestasis. *Hepatology* **29**:1003–6.

15. Zylicz Z, Smits C, Krajnik M. (1998). Paroxetine for pruritus in advanced cancer. *J Pain Symptom Manage* **16**:121–4.

16. Hutchings HA, Eccles R. (1994). The opioid agonist codeine and antagonist naltrexone do not affect voluntary suppression of capsaicin induced cough in healthy subjects. *Eur Respir J* **7**:715–19.

17. Dicpinigaitis PV, Allusson VR, Baldanti A, Nalamati JR. (2001). Ethnic and gender differences in cough reflex sensitivity. *Respiration* **68**:480–2.

18. Dicpinigaitis PV, Rauf K. (1998). The influence of gender on cough reflex sensitivity. *Chest* **113**:1319–21.

19. Sumitra S, Yesudian P. (1993). Friction amyloidosis: a variant or an etiologic factor in amyloidosis cutis? *Int J Dermatol* **32**:422–3.

20. Kelly R. (1977). Dermatoses in geriatric patients. *Aust Fam Physician* **6**:36–44.

21. Hunter JA. (1985). Seventh age itch. *Br Med J (Clin Res Ed)* **291**:842.

22. Long CC, Marks R. (1992). Stratum corneum changes in patients with senile pruritus. *J Am Acad Dermatol* **27**:560–4.

23. Teofoli P, De Pita O, Frezzolini A, Lotti T. (1998). Antipruritic effect of oral cyclosporin A in essential senile pruritus. *Acta Derm Venereol* **78**:232.

24. Daly BM, Shuster S. (2000). Antipruritic action of thalidomide. *Acta Derm Venereol* **80**:24–5.

25. Bernhard JD. (1992). Phantom itch, pseudophantom itch, and senile pruritus. *Int J Dermatol* **31**:856–7.

26. Balin AK, Pratt LA. (1989). Physiological consequences of human skin aging. *Cutis* **43**:431–6.

27. Farkas J. (1982). Chronic shoe dermatitis from chromium tanned leather. *Contact Dermatitis* **8**:140.

28. Woodward DF, Nieves AL, Hawley SB, Joseph R, Merlino GF, Spada CS. (1995). The pruritogenic and inflammatory effects of prostanoids in the conjunctiva. *J Ocul Pharmacol Ther* **11**:339–47.

29. Chan L. (1989). Investigation and treatment of vaginal discharge and pruritus vulvae. *Singapore Med J* **30**:471–2.

30. Vincent C. (1999). Anorectal pain and irritation: anal fissure, levator syndrome, proctalgia fugax, and pruritus ani. *Prim Care* **26**:53–68.

31. Taniguchi S, Yamamoto N, Kono T, Hamada T. (1996). Generalized pruritus in anorexia nervosa. *Br J Dermatol* **134**:510–1.

32. Hejna M, Valencak J, Raderer M. (1999). Anal pruritus after cancer chemotherapy with gemcitabine. *N Engl J Med* **340**:655–6.

33. Hermens JM, Ebertz JM, Hanifin JM, Hirshman CA. (1985). Comparison of histamine release in human skin mast cells induced by morphine, fentanyl, and oxymorphone. *Anesthesiology* **62**:124–9.

34. Taleb N, Geahchan N, Ghosn M, Brihi E, Sacre P. (1988). Vulvar pruritus after high-dose dexamethasone. *Eur J Cancer Clin Oncol* **24**:495.

35. Schlaepfer WW. (1968). Ultrastructural and histochemical studies of a primary sensory neuropathy in rats produced by chronic lead intoxication. *J Neuropathol Exp Neurol* **27**:111–2.

36. Nakada S, Saito H, Imura N. (1981). Effect of methylmercury and inorganic mercury on the nerve growth factor-induced neurite outgrowth in chick embryonic sensory ganglia. *Toxicol Lett* **8**:23–8.

37. Weiss JJ, Thompson GR, Lazaro R. (1982). Gold toxicity presenting as peripheral neuropathy. *Clin Rheumatol* **1**:285–9.

38. Singer R, Valciukas JA, Lilis R. (1983). Lead exposure and nerve conduction velocity: the differential time course of sensory and motor nerve effects. *Neurotoxicology* **4**:193–202.

39. Cousins MJ, Mather LE. (1984). Intrathecal and epidural administration of opioids. *Anesthesiology* **61**:276–310.

40. Bellinger DC, Needleman HL, Leviton A, Waternaux C, Rabinowitz MB, Nichols ML. (1984). Early sensory-motor development and prenatal exposure to lead. *Neurobehav Toxicol Teratol* **6**:387–402.

41. Arvidson B, Arvidsson J. (1990). Retrograde axonal transport of mercury in primary sensory neurons innervating the tooth pulp in the rat. *Neurosci Lett* **115**:29–32.

42. Hadfield-Law L. (2000). Scratching the itch: management of scabies in A & E. *Accid Emerg Nurs* **8**:230–2.

43. Wilson AD, Harwood LJ, Bjornsdottir S, Marti E, Day MJ. (2001). Detection of IgG and IgE serum antibodies to Culicoides salivary gland antigens in horses with insect dermal hypersensitivity (sweet itch). *Equine Vet J* **33**:707–13.

44. Andoh T, Katsube N, Maruyama M, Kuraishi Y. (2001). Involvement of leukotriene B(4) in substance P-induced itch-associated response in mice. *J Invest Dermatol* **117**:1621–6.

45. Zhai H, Simion FA, Abrutyn E, Koehler AM, Maibach HI. (2002). Screening topical antipruritics: a histamine-induced itch human model. *Skin Pharmacol Appl Skin Physiol* **15**:213–17.

46. Forsell M, Marcusson JA, Carlmark B, Johansson O. (1997). Analysis of the metal content of *in vivo*-fixed dental alloys by means of a simple office procedure. *Swed Dent J* **21**:161–8.

47. Beare JM. (1976). Generalized pruritus. A study of 43 cases. *Clin Exp Dermatol* **1**:343–52.

48. Gilchrest BA. (1982). Pruritus: pathogenesis, therapy, and significance in systemic disease states. *Arch Intern Med* **142**:101–5.

49. Kantor GR, Lookingbill DP. (1983). Generalized pruritus and systemic disease. *J Am Acad Dermatol* **9**:375–82.

50. Greaves MW. (1992). Itching—research has barely scratched the surface. *N Engl J Med* **326**:1016–17.

51. Diamond S, Prager J, Freitag FG. (1986). Diet and headache. Is there a link? *Postgrad Med* **79**:279–86.

52. Lewis J, Lieberman P, Treadwell G, Erffmeyer J. (1981). Exercise-induced urticaria, angioedema, and anaphylactoid episodes. *J Allergy Clin Immunol* **68**:432–7.

53. Novey HS, Fairshter RD, Salness K, Simon RA, Curd JG. (1983). Postprandial exercise-induced anaphylaxis. *J Allergy Clin Immunol* **71**:498–504.

54. Silvers WS. (1992). Exercise-induced allergies: the role of histamine release. *Ann Allergy* **68**:58–63.

55. Lun X, Rong L. (2000). Twenty-five cases of intractable cutaneous pruritus treated by auricular acupuncture. *J Tradit Chin Med* **20**:287–8.

56. Thomsen JS, Petersen MB, Benfeldt E, Jensen SB, Serup J. (2001). Scratch induction in the rat by intradermal serotonin: a model for pruritus. *Acta Derm Venereol* **81**:250–4.

57. Haustein UF. (1990). Adrenergic urticaria and adrenergic pruritus. *Acta Derm Venereol* **70**:82–4.

58. du Peloux Menage H, Greaves MW. (1995). Aquagenic pruritus. *Semin Dermatol* **14**:313–16.

59. Abdel-Naser MB, Gollnick H, Orfanos CE. (1993). Aquagenic pruritus as a presenting symptom of polycythemia vera. *Dermatology* **187**:130–3.

60. Rosenbaum M. (1988). Pruritus of unknown origin. *Hosp Pract* (*Off Ed*) **23**:19–22, 24, 26.

61. Smith PF, Corelli RL. (1997). Doxepin in the management of pruritus associated with allergic cutaneous reactions. *Ann Pharmacother* **31**:633–5.

62. Zylicz Z, Krajnik M. (1999). Codeine for pruritus in primary biliary cirrhosis. *Lancet* **353**:813.

63. Zirwas MJ, Seraly MP. (2001). Pruritus of unknown origin: a retrospective study. *J Am Acad Dermatol* **45**:892–6.

64. Jimenez-Alonso J, Tercedor J, Reche I. (2000). Antimalarial drugs and pruritus in patients with lupus erythematosus. *Acta Derm Venereol* **80**:458.

4

Measurement of scratching activity

E. Anthony Jones, Hugo Molenaar, and Nora V. Bergasa

Problems in evaluating treatments for pruritus

Although data on the pathophysiology of cholestasis may be obtained from animal models,[1–3] to obtain definitive insights into the pathogenesis of the pruritus of cholestasis and to demonstrate the efficacy of treatments for this condition, clinical studies are necessary. In clinical trials of drugs for the pruritus of cholestasis, for example, it is necessary to determine whether an amelioration of pruritus is due to a spontaneous pathophysiological change, or to a placebo or therapeutic effect. In this context, the design of such trials should, if possible, be prospective, randomized, double-blind, and placebo-controlled.

Pruritus is an intrinsically subjective perception; it cannot be quantitated directly. Although application of visual analogue scores of the perception of pruritus can be used to generate numbers, such data represent an inadequate and unreliable method of quantifying the pruritus of cholestasis. The clinical application of visual analogue scales (VAS) has been critically reviewed by MacCormack et al.[4] Potential problems include:

- a trimodal distribution of data with clusters at the midpoint and extremes of the visual analogue scales;
- interpatient variability in marking the scales;
- the requirement of an ability to transform a complex subjective experience into a visuospatial display (involving perceptual judgement and accuracy);
- a variety of factors that contribute to respondent error (e.g. age, ability to think abstractly, mental organization, perceptual skills);

- a desire to look at how scales were marked on previous occasions;
- early use of the maximum value, which precludes subsequent accurate scoring of a greater perception.

Accordingly, subjective data on the perception of pruritus in cholestatic patients are likely to be unreliable and of uncertain meaning.[4] This prediction is supported by practical experience with the application of VAS in clinical trials of new therapies for the pruritus of cholestasis. A basic requirement of well designed therapeutic trials is that a meaningful objective reliable quantitative efficacy end-point be incorporated into their design.

Scratching activity, in the context of the pruritus of cholestasis, can be defined as the behavioural consequence of this complication of cholestasis. In contrast to pruritus, scratching activity can be quantitated. Thus, the problems inherent in assessing the severity of the subjective perception of pruritus may be obviated by objectively quantifying scratching activity. While scratching activity has been claimed to correlate strongly with itching,[5] the severity of the perception of the pruritus of cholestasis, as described subjectively by patients, does not necessarily correlate closely with scratching activity.[4, 6, 7] Initial attempts to quantitate scratching activity involved the application of sophisticated limb and hand movement meters.[8, 9] The development of these pioneer methods reflected the need to apply objective quantitative methods in clinical studies of pruritus. Unfortunately, measurements of limb and hand movements record activities in addition to scratching activity. Ideally, scratching activity should be quantitated independent of extraneous arm and hand movements.

Application of piezo-film technology to measure scratching activity

The first monitoring system designed to quantitate scratching activity independent of limb movements comprised a vibration (scratch) transducer consisting of a piece of piezoelectric film (polyvinylidene fluoride, PVDF), an FM transmitter and receiver, a custom-made signal processor, and a personal computer (Fig. 4.1).[10]

The PVDF film was 28 μm thick and was supplied with metallization on both sides—a sputtered aluminium–nickel alloy to create an electrical contact to the film. Two components were attached to an arm of the patient: (1) the transducer was glued to the nail of the middle finger of the dominant hand with a removable medical-grade adhesive, reinforced

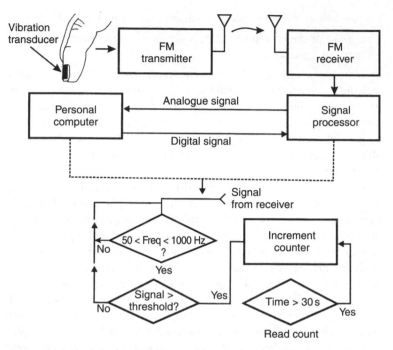

Fig. 4.1 Block diagram of the prototypic scratching activity monitoring system with a flow chart of the signal-processing scheme. Reproduced with permission from (10).

with adhesive tape; (2) a battery-powered transmitter was attached to the corresponding upper arm. The transducer acts as a contact microphone on the finger nail. When the finger nail vibrates as it traverses the skin in the act of scratching, it induces bends (physical strain) in the piezo-film that result in generating an electrical signal. The signal from the film is telemetered to a receiver located several metres away from the patient. The telemetry system is based on an FM wireless microphone system operating at a frequency (e.g. 49.89 MHz) that is free from interference.

The main component of the system, represented in the lower portion of Fig. 4.1, is a signal processor designed to produce a signal proportional to the duration and intensity of scratching. The signal processor is a frequency counter incorporating a threshold detector and a bandpass filter to inhibit extraneous counts not directly related to scratching. The threshold detector discriminates between gentle rubbing and robust scratching by imposing the requirement that the vibration amplitude of the transducer exceed a predetermined level. This level was determined by analysing chart-recorded signals from a normal volunteer who purposely and randomly performed an exhaustive number of manoeuvres with his fingers, hand, and arm while intermixing episodes of scratching. The threshold level was adjusted such that approximately 90% of the scratch signal was captured, while the signal associated with gentle rubbing or incidental contact with the sensor was excluded.

The chosen upper and lower cut-off frequencies of the analogue band-pass filter were based on Fourier analysis of the raw signal from the PVDF film obtained during scratching. This analysis revealed that the power of the signal associated with scratching was concentrated in a band of frequencies between 50 Hz and 1 kHz (Fig. 4.2). An analogue comparator with hysteresis generates a pulse that increments each time the counter voltage (positive or negative) from the bandpass filter exceeds the threshold. The personal computer via an I/O port on an A/D converter interface card generates a latch-reset pulse every 30 seconds that latches the total count value. The D/A converter yields an analogue voltage proportional to the number of counts occurring during each consecutive 30-second interval. Count values are read by the computer and stored on disk for later analysis.

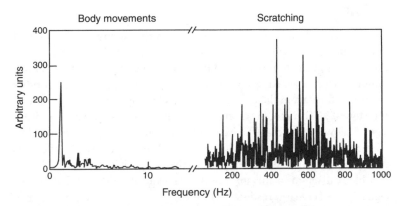

Fig. 4.2 Power spectrum obtained by Fourier analysis of demodulated signals from the piezo-film scratch transducer as a patient scratches with the finger nail bearing the transducer. The frequencies generated by gross body movements are < 50 Hz and those generated by the scratching finger nail are between 50 and 1000 Hz. Reproduced with permission from (10).

To avoid the use of microconductor cables, the count value was converted to an analogue voltage for input to the computer. The A/D converter on the DAS16 converts the analogue voltage into a digital number that is directly proportional to the incoming signal level. This number, which is proportional to the number of times that the filtered signal exceeds the preset threshold during a 30-second period, has been designated a scratching activity index.

Verification that the measured scratching activity index is a genuine representation of scratching activity was accomplished by both videotapes and independent visual observations. Practical problems in operating this monitoring system and their solution are discussed by Talbot *et al.*[10] The system has been successfully applied to provide an objective quantitative efficacy end-point in four trials of the efficacy of opiate antagonists in the management of the pruritus of cholestasis.[6, 7, 11, 12]

The main disadvantage of this prototypic device is that the patient is required to be confined to a hospital room (near the receiver) throughout the period of the recording, and hence is not in his or her normal environment. This disadvantage may be important as the pruritus may be influenced by a change of environment.

An improved device for measuring scratching activity

The problem of confining a patient to a room throughout the duration of a recording of scratching activity has been overcome by processing and storing the signals from the transducer over a predetermined interval in a computer chip attached to the patient's body. At the end of the period of recording, the data in the chip can be unloaded into a personal computer and stored.[13] This modification of the monitoring system has the advantage of allowing scratching activity to be recorded while the patient is in a normal environment, such as home or work-place. Thus, any effects of change of environment on scratching activity are obviated.

A block diagram of this improved data acquisition device is shown in Fig. 4.3. The scratch transducer also incorporates a piezo-element that is attached to a finger nail. Electrical signals from the transducer are fed through a filter/amplifier. The bandpass filter, with its −3 dB points at 70 Hz and 1200 Hz, removes artefacts caused by natural movements of the hand and arm, by excluding data with a frequency of < 70 Hz (Fig. 4.4). The signal coming from the filter is led to an adjustable threshold

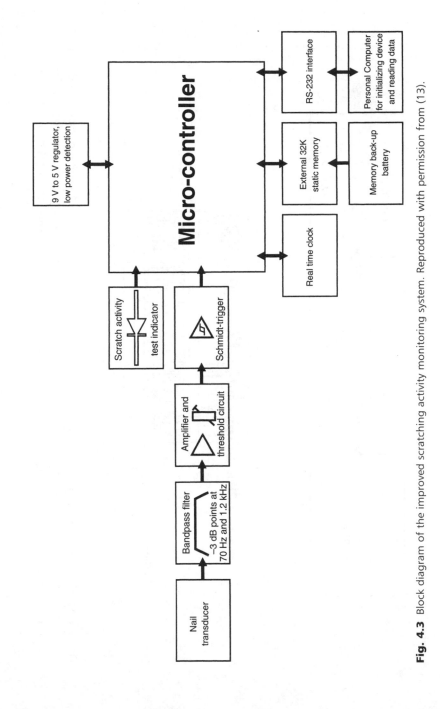

Fig. 4.3 Block diagram of the improved scratching activity monitoring system. Reproduced with permission from (13).

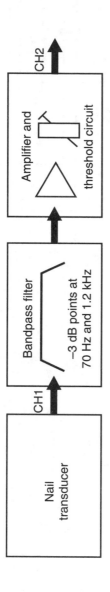

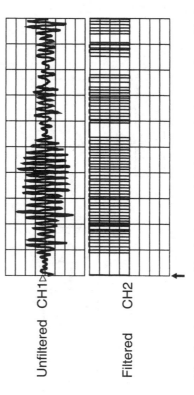

Fig. 4.4 Nature of the signals generated by the improved device attached to a patient with the pruritus of cholestasis during the act of scratching with the finger nail bearing the scratch transducer. CH1, unfiltered signal from the scratch transducer; CH2, filtered signal coming from the amplifier and threshold circuit. Reproduced with permission from (13).

circuit. The output of the circuit is connected directly to a 74HCT132 Schmitt-trigger gate, the output of which is led to a microcontroller.

A personal computer can be connected to the microprocessor to initialize the datalogger to record data during a programmed time interval and to unload the data after a period of recording. During periods of recording, data are temporarily stored in a 32k static RAM. To relate data to time, a real time clock, which communicates with the microcontroller via a IC2 bus, is added. Five volt power is derived from a standard 9 V battery. A switched step-down converter is used to maintain the supply voltage at 5 V until the battery power fails. A backup for the static RAM is given by a memcap of 0.1 F. The standard 9 V battery enables data to be recorded continuously for at least 48 hours. The electronic components and battery fit into a small box ($9.6 \times 6.1 \times 2.3$ cm). The complete device, with battery, weighs 170 g.

The piezo-element was secured at one end of a stainless-steel tube (length about 18 mm; diameter 4 mm) with epoxy, leaving the other end free to vibrate. The tube was closed at one end with epoxy and at the other end it was occluded by compressing the metal. The transducer is glued to the surface of the middle fingernail of the dominant hand with a cyano-acrylate gel. The wire connecting the transducer to the device is worn under the patient's clothing.

The firmware for the device and the software for the scratching-activity recording program were written in C. The start time and duration of a new period of measurement can be set at will. In practice, an interval of 30 seconds was chosen for each consecutive count, and a period of 24 hours was chosen as the total duration of a period of recording. The numbers generated each 30 seconds represent an activity tag or vibration count that reflects the intensity of scratching and constitutes an objective quantitative index of scratching activity. Typical scratching activity data obtained using this device are shown in Fig. 4.5. The practical application of the device is discussed in greater detail by Molenaar et al.[13]

Conclusions

• Monitoring systems have been designed to generate a quantitative index of scratching activity that is independent of arm or hand movements.

• These systems, which have been validated, depend on the application of piezo-film technology to measure the vibrations of a fingernail as it traverses the skin in the act of scratching.

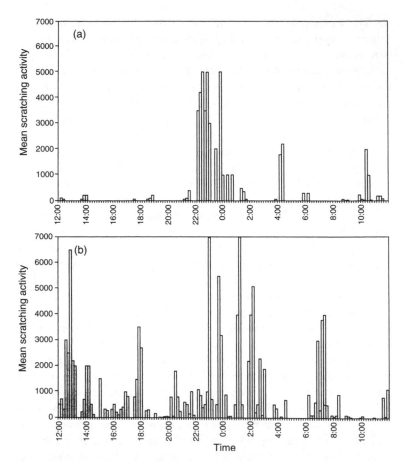

Fig. 4.5 Representative 24-hour plots of scratching activity data in a patient with the pruritus of cholestasis obtained using the improved device.
(a) During treatment with an experimental drug for the pruritus of cholestasis.
(b) During treatment with a placebo. Reproduced with permission from (13).

- They can be applied to provide an objective quantitative efficacy end-point in trials of therapies, not only for pruritus associated with cholestasis, but for pruritus of any cause.
- Processing and storing signals from a scratch transducer in a computer chip attached to the patient's body enables scratching activity to be recorded in ambulant patients.

References

1. Bergasa NV, Rothman RB, Vergalla J, Xu H, Swain MG, Jones EA. (1992). Central mu-opioid receptors are down-regulated in a rat model of cholestasis. *J Hepatol* **15**:220–4.

2. Swain MG, Rothman RB, Xu H, Vergalla J, Bergasa NV, Jones EA. (1992). Endogenous opioids accumulate in plasma in a rat model of acute cholestasis. *Gastroenterology* **103**:630–5.

3. Bergasa NV, Alling DW, Vergalla J, Jones EA. (1994). Cholestasis in the male rat is associated with naloxone-reversible antinociception. *J Hepatol* **20**:85–90.

4. McCormack HM, Horne DJ, Sheather S. (1988). Clinical applications of visual analogue scales: a critical review. *Psychol Med* **18**:1007–19.

5. Shelly WB, Arthur RP. (1957). The neurohistology and neurophysiology of the itch sensation in man. *AMA Arch Dermatol* **76**:296–323.

6. Bergasa NV, Alling DW, Talbot TL, Wells MC, Jones EA. (1999). Oral nalmefene therapy reduces scratching activity due to the pruritus of cholestasis: a controlled study. *J Am Acad Dermatol* **41**:431–4.

7. Bergasa NV, Talbot TL, Alling DW, et al. (1992). A controlled trial of naloxone infusions for the pruritus of chronic cholestasis. *Gastroenterology* **102**:544–9.

8. Felix R, Shuster S. (1975). A new method for the measurement of itch and the response to treatment. *Br J Dermatol* **93**:303–12.

9. Summerfield JA, Welch ME. (1980). The measurement of itch with sensitive limb movement meters. *Br J Dermatol* **103**:275–81.

10. Talbot TL, Schmitt JM, Bergasa NV, Jones EA, Walker EC. (1991). Application of piezo film technology for the quantitative assessment of pruritus. *Biomed Instrum Technol* **25**:400–3.

11. Bergasa NV, Alling DW, Talbot TL, et al. (1995). Effects of naloxone infusions in patients with the pruritus of cholestasis. A double-blind, randomized, controlled trial. *Ann Intern Med* **123**:161–7.

12. Bergasa NV, Schmitt JM, Talbot TL, et al. (1998). Open-label trial of oral nalmefene therapy for the pruritus of cholestasis. *Hepatology* **27**:679–84.

13. Molenaar HA, Oosting J, Jones EA. (1998). Improved device for measuring scratching activity in patients with pruritus. *Med Biol Eng Comput* **36**:220–4.

5

The pruritus of cholestasis and the opioid neurotransmitter system

E. Anthony Jones and Nora V. Bergasa

Definition and prevalence

Pruritus is experienced by about 80% of jaundiced patients. It is a presenting symptom in 25–70% of patients with chronic cholestatic liver diseases, such as primary biliary cirrhosis, and is experienced by at least 80% of patients during the course of these diseases.[1–5] Pruritus is a presenting symptom in approximately 5% of patients with the non-cholestatic liver disease, chronic hepatitis C.[6] Rarely, pruritus complicates other non-cholestatic liver disorders, such as chronic hepatitis B and chronic alcoholic liver disease.

Clinical presentation

Cholestasis is the syndrome that arises as a consequence of impaired bile secretion and/or flow, which leads to the regurgitation of components of bile into plasma and is associated with an increase in serum alkaline phosphatase levels. This form of pruritus is not effectively eased by scratching. There is no evidence of a primary pruritic skin lesion, but lesions secondary to scratching, such as excoriations or *prurigo nodularis*, may develop. In many patients with the pruritus of cholestasis the symptom is so distressing that it interferes with normal activities. It can cause severe sleep deprivation. Unrelieved pruritus of cholestasis can lead to suicidal ideation and can be an indication for liver transplantation, irrespective of evidence of hepatic decompensation or indices of prognosis of the underlying liver disease.[7]

Pathogenesis

The pathogenesis of the pruritus of cholestasis is unknown.[8] Pruritus tends to subside rapidly if the cause of cholestasis is removed, for example, when large duct biliary obstruction is relieved by stenting. However, a decrease in itching in a cholestatic patient does not always imply a decrease in the severity of cholestasis and/or improvement in hepatocellular function. In some patients with chronic progressive cholestatic liver diseases, itching may subside spontaneously without any obvious change in the severity of the cholestasis as the disease progresses and chronic hepatocellular failure supervenes. This clinical observation suggests that a substance(s) that contributes, directly or indirectly, to the pruritus of cholestasis is synthesized by the cholestatic liver.

The concept of peripherally acting pruritogens

For decades it was assumed that the pruritus of cholestasis arises peripherally as a consequence of interactions between nerve endings in the skin and one or more substances that accumulate systemically as a result of their impaired biliary secretion. Hypotheses of pathogenesis have often been based on correlations between subjective assessments of pruritus and levels of specific substances in plasma or interstitial fluid of the skin. However, for a correlation to have potential pathogenic relevance, it is necessary to show that the substance measured can induce neurophysiological changes that mediate pruritus. This requirement has not been fulfilled for putative peripherally acting pruritogens in cholestatic patients (e.g. bile acids).[8]

Therapy based on the assumption of peripherally acting pruritogens

The presumed rationale for most commonly used therapies for the pruritus of cholestasis appears to be to reduce the concentrations of putative pruritogens at nerve endings in the skin. Examples of such therapeutic agents include anion exchange resins, such as colestyramine and colestipol, and hepatic enzyme-inducing drugs, such as rifampicin, phenobarbital, and flumecinol.[8] The same rationale applies to invasive approaches to management, such as plasmapheresis, charcoal haemoperfusion, and partial external diversion of bile.[8] The fact that such measures have been tried indicates that more conventional therapeutic modalities are not efficacious. The nature of any potentially relevant substance has not been identified in trials of empirical therapies that affect the metabolism of many compounds.

H_1-antihistamines are often administered to patients with the pruritus of cholestasis, but have not been shown to be efficacious. Sedatives, such as phenobarbital, benzodiazepines, and antihistamines, may have a non-specific beneficial effect. Sedation may facilitate work during the day by improving sleep at night. On the other hand, sedation may impair activities that require concentration, such as driving and operating machinery. Among miscellaneous therapies that have been tried are phototherapy, lidocaine, androgens, hydroxyethylrutosides, and ursodeoxycholic acid.[8] None has a sound rationale and none has been shown to be efficacious in a randomized controlled trial.

Certain empirical therapies continue to be widely used in practice. There is a consensus that an appreciable proportion of patients with chronic cholestatic liver disease experience an amelioration of pruritus when treated with an anion exchange resin or rifampicin, and this consensus is supported by subjective data from double-blind randomized controlled trials.[9–11]

Theoretically, a treatment that reverses cholestasis would also be expected to reverse the consequences of cholestasis that mediate pruritus. However, drugs that are believed to have this property, for example, S-adenosyl-methionine[12] and ursodeoxycholic acid,[13] have not been shown to be consistently efficacious.

The concept of pruritus of central origin

The assumption that the primary event in the initiation of the pruritus of cholestasis is peripheral within the skin is not supported by convincing data. Consequently, it is necessary to consider whether non-peripheral pruritogenic events may contribute to this form of pruritus. The association of certain neurological and psychiatric diseases with pruritus, in the absence of any skin lesion, indicates that pruritus can arise centrally in the brain.[14, 15] However, there is no evidence that any neurological or psychiatric defect is consistently a component of the syndrome of cholestasis.

In this context a specific mechanism of pruritus of central origin, suggested by pharmacology texts, is of potential interest. This mechanism appears to involve the interaction between opioid agonists, such as morphine, and opioid receptors in the central nervous system (CNS). In particular, 'pruritus may, in part, involve effects of opioids on neurons, since it is provoked by opioids that do not release histamine and is quickly abolished by small doses of the opioid antagonist, naloxone'[16] and 'central modulators of pruritus, such as morphine, cause itch. . .by acting on central opioid receptors'.[15] Indeed, 'itching' has been reported to be an effect of morphine on the central nervous system.[17] Other opioid agonists have also been implicated in the mediation of pruritus.[18]

The opioid neurotransmitter system

In considering whether opioid-induced pruritus might have any implications for the pruritus of cholestasis, it is necessary to distinguish the systemic effects of opioids from their local effects near injection sites. Local effects, after intradermal injection, include histamine release, urticaria, and local pruritus that is not reversed by naloxone and hence is not mediated by opioid receptors.[16] These local effects do not appear to be relevant to the pruritus of cholestasis. Both increased central opioidergic tone and generalized pruritus are systemic effects of opioids,[16] and it is the association of increased central opioidergic tone with pruritus that may have relevance to the pathogenesis of the pruritus of cholestasis. Indeed, it has been proposed that increased opioidergic neurotransmission/neuromodulation (tone) in the CNS contributes to the pruritus of cholestasis.[19] This hypothesis would be strongly supported if the following could be demonstrated.

* Opioid receptor ligands with agonist properties mediate pruritus by a central mechanism.
* Opioid-mediated neurotransmission/neuromodulation (tone) in the CNS is increased in cholestasis.
* The pruritus of cholestasis can be reversed (at least partially) by opioid antagonists.

Opioid agonists and pruritus of central origin

When morphine (0.2–0.5 mg/kg) is injected intracisternally into cats, violent scratching activity is induced that lasts for up to 90 minutes.[20] Furthermore, microinjections of morphine (1–10 μg) or the opioid agonist ligand (D-Ala^2-N-Me-Phe^4-Gly-ol^5)-enkephalin (but not saline) into the medullary dorsal horn of monkeys (*Macaca fasicularis*) induces dose-dependent facial scratching activity that is abolished by naloxone.[21] These observations indicate that opioid agonists induce opioid receptor-mediated scratching activity of central origin.

The status of the opioid system in cholestasis

Five distinct lines of evidence are consistent with opioidergic tone being increased in cholestasis.

1. In patients with chronic cholestatic liver disease, 5 mg of the potent opioid antagonist, nalmefene, consistently induces an abrupt reaction with many features in common with the classical withdrawal reaction of opioid addiction (Box 5.1). The reaction is transient, usually subsiding spontaneously after 2–3 days in spite of continued administration of nalmefene. This reaction does not occur when nalmefene is administered even in higher doses to normal subjects.[22]

2. Rats with cholestasis due to bile duct resection exhibit antinociception (analgesia) that is stereoselectively reversed by naloxone and, hence, is mediated by opioid receptors. In contrast, the rat model of thioacetamide-induced acute hepatocellular necrosis does not exhibit naloxone-reversible antinociception.[23]

3. Total opioid activity in plasma is increased in a rat model of cholestasis and the concentrations of individual endogenous opioid agonists are elevated in the plasma of rats and humans with cholestasis.[22, 24]

4. Plasma extracts from patients with the pruritus of cholestasis, but not extracts from non-pruritic cholestatic controls, induce naloxone-reversible facial scratching when micro-injected into the medullary dorsal horn of monkeys.[25] Thus, plasma of patients with the pruritus of cholestasis contains one or more substances that can induce central opioid receptor-mediated scratching activity.

5. In the rat model of cholestasis due to bile duct resection, μ-opioid receptors in the brain are downregulated,[26] possibly due to changes in

Box 5.1 Reaction in patients with chronic cholestasis precipitated by a potent opioid antagonist[22]

- Anorexia
- Nausea
- Colicky abdominal pain
- Increase in systolic and diastolic blood pressure
- Slow pulse
- Pallor
- Cool skin
- Mood changes
- Visual and auditory hallucinations

opioid receptor kinetics in response to increased availability of endogenous opioids at opioid receptors.

Taken together these five diverse lines of evidence strongly suggest that central opioidergic tone is increased in cholestasis.

Modulation of the pruritus of cholestasis by opioid antagonists

Using subjective methods of assessment:

1. A subcutaneous injection of naloxone was reported in 1979 to induce a dramatic amelioration of intractable pruritus in a patient with primary biliary cirrhosis, whereas an injection of saline appeared to have no effect.[27]

2. The oral administration of nalmefene to 9 patients with primary biliary cirrhosis was reported to be associated with substantial ameliorations of pruritus, which appeared to be sustained over a 6-month period of drug administration.[22]

3. Orally administered naltrexone appeared to be more efficacious than a placebo in ameliorating pruritus in patients with chronic cholestatic liver disease.[28]

These subjective findings suggest that opioid antagonists may mediate a beneficial effect in patients with the pruritus of cholestasis. Using a monitoring system that objectively quantitates scratching activity independent of limb movements,[29] scratching activity in patients with pruritus due to chronic cholestatic liver diseases was shown to be significantly less during naloxone infusions than during placebo infusions in two controlled trials (Fig. 5.1).[30, 31] Furthermore, in one of these trials, which had a randomized, double-blind design, the mean visual analogue score of the perception of pruritus was significantly less during naloxone infusions than during placebo infusions.[31]

The results of these studies indicate that in patients with the pruritus of cholestasis an opioid antagonist can not only reduce scratching activity, but can probably also decrease the perception of pruritus.

Thus, both clinical and experimental findings appear to provide strong support for the hypothesis that altered opioidergic tone in the CNS contributes to the pathogenesis of the pruritus of cholestasis. Accordingly, the pathogenic mechanisms involved in the mediation of the pruritus of cholestasis would be expected to include central neuronal events induced

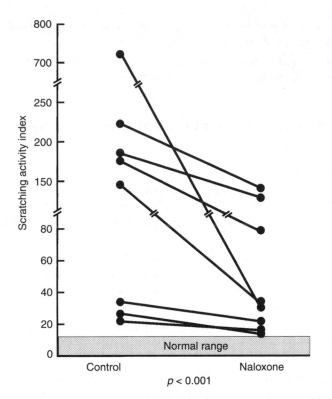

Fig. 5.1 Mean hourly scratching activity during 24 hour infusions of either naloxone or placebo in 8 patients with primary biliary cirrhosis. The decrease in scratching activity associated with the administration of naloxone (0.2 µg/kg/min) ranges from 29 to 96% (mean 50%, $p < 0.001$). (Reproduced with permission from (30).)

by opioid agonist ligand/receptor interactions (e.g. activation of neuronal G-proteins and ion channels) that lead to stimulation of the motor pathways that mediate scratching activity. Whether opioid receptors on peripheral neurons are involved in the pathogenesis of the pruritus of cholestasis is unknown.

Currently available data do not indicate which endogenous opioid receptor ligands may be responsible for contributing to pruritus in cholestatic patients, or which opioid antagonists may be optimal for use in the short- or long-term treatment of this condition. Furthermore, they do not indicate whether the factors responsible for increased opioidergic tone in cholestasis originate peripherally or centrally. Only interactions between certain opioid peptides and certain opioid receptor subtypes may be relevant to the pruritus of cholestasis. Both the nature and the source of the endogenous opioids involved in the pruritus of cholestasis are currently unknown, but one source may be the cholestatic liver itself.[32] There may be increased plasma-to-brain transfer of endogenous opioid peptides in cholestasis[33] due to their accumulation in plasma,[22, 24] and this process would be facilitated by their amphoteric properties. However, the potential relevance of this phenomenon to the pathogenesis of the pruritus of cholestasis remains to be determined.

The observation that rifampicin induces an opioid withdrawal syndrome in patients on maintenance doses of methadone[34] raises the possibility that apparent ameliorations of the pruritus of cholestasis induced by rifampicin[9–11] may be attributable to an effect of rifampicin on the opioid neurotransmitter system, which leads to a decrease in opioidergic tone. Apparent ameliorations of the pruritus of cholestasis after the administration of propofol[35, 36] may also be attributable to a modulation of opioidergic tone.

Potential therapeutic implications of opioid antagonists

The available data on the effects of opioid antagonists on the pruritus of cholestasis suggest that parenterally administered naloxone may have a place in the emergency treatment of a severe exacerbation of the pruritus of cholestasis[30, 31] and that nalmefene may have a place in long-term management of pruritus in patients with chronic cholestatic liver diseases.[22] These tentative inferences are supported by a comparison of the properties of these two opioid antagonists. In particular, when compared to naloxone, nalmefene is substantially more bioavailable when given by mouth, it has a more potent antagonist action at opioid receptors, and it is metabolized more slowly, resulting in a longer plasma half-life.[37] Both an open-label trial[37] and a placebo-controlled trial,[38] in which scratching activity was quantitated, suggest that nalmefene may indeed be useful for the long-term control of the pruritus of cholestasis (Figs 5.2 and 5.3). Naltrexone may be an efficacious alternative to nalmefene in this context.[28]

While recent findings indicate that opioid antagonists may be efficacious in ameliorating the pruritus of cholestasis, some patients with severe pruritus associated with cholestatic disorders have not experienced substantial relief from the perception of pruritus over the short term, following

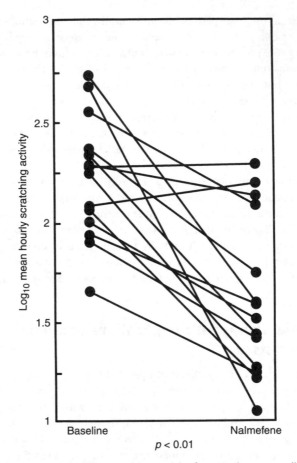

Fig. 5.2 Log_{10} mean hourly scratching activity from 24 hour recordings in patients with the pruritus of cholestasis before and during treatment with orally-administered nalmefene.
(Reproduced with permission from (37).)

administration of an opioid antagonist. However, quality dose–response data are sparse.

The possibility of precipitating an opioid withdrawal-like syndrome when initiating long-term treatment with an orally bioavailable opioid antagonist is a clinically significant issue.[22, 39–42] It may be possible to avoid the precipitation of such a reaction by first infusing naloxone, initially at a low subtherapeutic dose,[39] and, subsequently, gradually increasing the

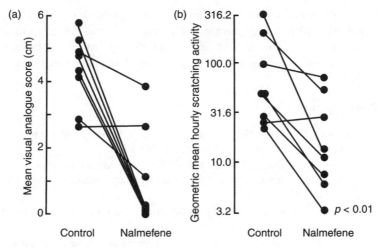

Fig. 5.3 Effects of randomized blinded oral administration of nalmefene to 8 patients with chronic cholestatic liver disease. (a) Mean visual analogue scores of the perception of pruritus during control periods (baseline and/or placebo) and during nalmefene therapy. (b) Geometric mean hourly scratching activity during control periods (baseline and/or placebo) and during nalmefene therapy.
(Reproduced with permission from (38).)

infusion rate to one within the therapeutic range,[30] before beginning oral administration of an opioid antagonist.[39–42]

Liver transplantation for intractable pruritus should not be undertaken before an adequate trial of opioid antagonist therapy.[40]

Conclusions

- Increased central opioidergic neurotransmission/neuromodulation (tone) is a component of the pathophysiology of cholestasis and contributes to the mediation of the pruritus that complicates this syndrome.

- The pruritus of cholestasis can be ameliorated by the administration of opioid antagonists. Those that are bioavailable when given orally and that readily cross the blood–brain barrier, for example, naltrexone and nalmefene, have potential for the long-term management of the pruritus of cholestasis.

- Administration of an orally bioavailable opioid antagonist to a cholestasic patient may precipitate an opioid withdrawal-like reaction. Such reactions can be avoided by cautiously infusing naloxone intravenously before giving the first oral dose of an opioid antagonist.

References

1. Sherlock S, Scheuer PJ. (1973). The presentation and diagnosis of 100 patients with primary biliary cirrhosis. *N Engl J Med* **289**:674–8.

2. Fleming CR, Ludwig J, Dickson ER. (1978). Asymptomatic primary biliary cirrhosis. Presentation, histology, and results with D-penicillamine. *Mayo Clin Proc* **53**:587–93.

3. James O, Macklon AF, Watson AJ. (1981). Primary biliary cirrhosis—a revised clinical spectrum. *Lancet* **1**:1278–81.

4. Jeffrey GP, Reed WD, Shilkin KB. (1990). Primary biliary cirrhosis: clinico-pathological characteristics and outcome. *J Gastroenterol Hepatol* **5**:639–45.

5. Brenard R, Degos F, Degott C, Lassoued K, Benhamou JP. (1990). Primary biliary cirrhosis: current modes of presentation. Clinical, biochemical, immunologic and histologic study of 206 patients seen from 1978 to 1988. *Gastroenterol Clin Biol* **14**:307–12.

6. Chia SC, Bergasa NV, Kleiner DE, Goodman Z, Hoofnagle JH, Di Bisceglie AM. (1998). Pruritus as a presenting symptom of chronic hepatitis C. *Dig Dis Sci* **43**:2177–83.

7. Elias E. (1993). Liver transplantation. *J R Coll Physicians Lond* **27**:224–32.

8. Bergasa NV, Jones EA. (1991). Management of the pruritus of cholestasis: potential role of opiate antagonists. *Am J Gastroenterol* **86**:1404–12.

9. Ghent CN, Carruthers SG. (1988). Treatment of pruritus in primary biliary cirrhosis with rifampin. Results of a double-blind, crossover, randomized trial. *Gastroenterology* **94**:488–93.

10. Cynamon HA, Andres JM, Iafrate RP. (1990). Rifampin relieves pruritus in children with cholestatic liver disease. *Gastroenterology* **98**:1013–16.

11. Bachs L, Pares A, Elena M, Piera C, Rodes J. (1989). Comparison of rifampicin with phenobarbitone for treatment of pruritus in biliary cirrhosis. *Lancet* **1**:574–6.

12. Frezza M, Surrenti C, Manzillo G, Fiaccadori F, Bortolini M, Di Padova C. (1990). Oral S-adenosylmethionine in the symptomatic treatment of intrahepatic cholestasis. A double-blind, placebo-controlled study. *Gastroenterology* **99**:211–15.

13. Poupon RE, Balkau B, Eschwege E, Poupon R. (1991). A multicenter, controlled trial of ursodiol for the treatment of primary biliary cirrhosis. UDCA-PBC Study Group. *N Engl J Med* **324**:1548–54.

14. Domonkos AN, Arnold HL, Odom RB. (1982). Pruritus and neurocutaneous dermatosis. In: Domonkos AN, Arnold HL, Richard B, Odom RB. (eds.), *Andrew's disease of the skin*, Philadelphia: WB Saunders, pp. 56–74.

15. Parker F. (1988) Skin diseases. In: Wijngaarden JB, Smith LH. (eds.), *Cecil textbook of medicine*, Philadelphia: WB Saunders, pp. 2300–53.

16. Jaffe JH, Martin WR. (1990) Opioid analgesics and antagonists. In: Gilman AG, Rail TW, Nies AS, Taylor P. (eds.), *Goodman and Gilman's the pharmacological basis of therapeutics*, New York: Pergamon Press. pp. 485–521.

17. Dollery C. (1991) Morphine. In: Dollery C. (ed.), *Therapeutic drugs*, New York: Churchill Livingstone, pp. M225–M233.

18. Jones EA, Bergasa NV. (1990). The pruritus of cholestasis: from bile acids to opiate agonists. *Hepatology* 11:884–7.

19. Bergasa NV, Jones EA. (1995). The pruritus of cholestasis: potential pathogenic and therapeutic implications of opioids. *Gastroenterology* 108:1582–8.

20. Koenigstein H. (1948). Experimental study of itch stimuli in animals. *Arch Dermatol Syph* 57:828–49.

21. Thomas DA, Williams GM, Iwata K, Kenshalo DR Jr, Dubner R. (1992). Effects of central administration of opioids on facial scratching in monkeys. *Brain Res* 585:315–17.

22. Thornton JR, Losowsky MS. (1988). Opioid peptides and primary biliary cirrhosis. *Br Med J* 297:1501–4.

23. Bergasa NV, Alling DW, Vergalla J, Jones EA. (1994). Cholestasis in the male rat is associated with naloxone-reversible antinociception. *J Hepatol* 20:85–90.

24. Swain MG, Rothman RB, Xu H, Vergalla J, Bergasa NV, Jones EA. (1992). Endogenous opioids accumulate in plasma in a rat model of acute cholestasis. *Gastroenterology* 103:630–5.

25. Bergasa NV, Thomas DA, Vergalla J, Turner ML, Jones EA. (1993). Plasma from patients with the pruritus of cholestasis induces opioid receptor-mediated scratching in monkeys. *Life Sci* 53:1253–7.

26. Bergasa NV, Rothman RB, Vergalla J, Xu H, Swain MG, Jones EA. (1992). Central mu-opioid receptors are down-regulated in a rat model of cholestasis. *J Hepatol* 15:220–4.

27. Bernstein JE, Swift R. (1979). Relief of intractable pruritus with naloxone. *Arch Dermatol* 115:1366–7.

28. Wolfhagen FH, Sternieri E, Hop WC, Vitale G, Bertolotti M, Van Buuren HR. (1997). Oral naltrexone treatment for cholestatic pruritus: a double-blind, placebo-controlled study. *Gastroenterology* 113:1264–9.

29. Talbot TL, Schmitt JM, Bergasa NV, Jones EA, Walker EC. (1991). Application of piezo film technology for the quantitative assessment of pruritus. *Biomed Instrum Technol* 25:400–3.

30. Bergasa NV, Talbot TL, Alling DW, et al. (1992). A controlled trial of naloxone infusions for the pruritus of chronic cholestasis. *Gastroenterology* **102**:544–9.

31. Bergasa NV, Alling DW, Talbot TL, et al. (1995). Effects of naloxone infusions in patients with the pruritus of cholestasis. A double-blind, randomized, controlled trial. *Ann Intern Med* **123**:161–7.

32. Bergasa NV, Sabol SL, Young WS 3rd, Kleiner DE, Jones EA. (1995). Cholestasis is associated with preproenkephalin mRNA expression in the adult rat liver. *Am J Physiol* **268**:G346–54.

33. Banks WA, Audus KL, Davis TP. (1992). Permeability of the blood–brain barrier to peptides: an approach to the development of therapeutically useful analogs. *Peptides* **13**:1289–94.

34. Kreek MJ, Garfield JW, Gutjahr CL, Giusti LM. (1976). Rifampin-induced methadone withdrawal. *N Engl J Med* **294**:1104–6.

35. Borgeat A, Wilder-Smith O, Mentha G, Huber O. (1992). Propofol and cholestatic pruritus. *Am J Gastroenterol* **87**:672–4.

36. Borgeat A, Wilder-Smith OH, Mentha G. (1993). Subhypnotic doses of propofol relieve pruritus associated with liver disease. *Gastroenterology* **104**:244–7.

37. Bergasa NV, Schmitt JM, Talbot TL, et al. (1998). Open-label trial of oral nalmefene therapy for the pruritus of cholestasis. *Hepatology* **27**:679–84.

38. Bergasa NV, Alling DW, Talbot TL, Wells MC, Jones EA. (1999). Oral nalmefene therapy reduces scratching activity due to the pruritus of cholestasis: a controlled study. *J Am Acad Dermatol* **41**:431–4.

39. Jones EA, Dekker LR. (2000). Florid opioid withdrawal-like reaction precipitated by naltrexone in a patient with chronic cholestasis. *Gastroenterology* **118**:431–2.

40. Neuberger J, Jones EA. (2001). Liver transplantation for intractable pruritus is contraindicated before an adequate trial of opiate antagonist therapy. *Eur J Gastroenterol Hepatol* **13**:1393–4.

41. Jones EA, Neuberger J, Bergasa NV. (2002). Opiate antagonist therapy for the pruritus of cholestasis: the avoidance of opioid withdrawal-like reactions. *QJM* **95**:547–52.

42. Jones EA. (2002). Trials of opiate antagonists for the pruritus of cholestasis: primary efficacy endpoints and opioid withdrawal-like reactions. *J Hepatol* **37**:863–5.

6

Uraemic pruritus

Jacek C. Szepietowski

Definition and synonyms

Pruritus was first linked to chronic renal failure by Chagrin and Keil in 1932.[1] Uraemic pruritus may be localized or generalized and is sometimes called dialysis pruritus. Pruritus is not a feature of acute renal failure. Before making a firm diagnosis, it is necessary to exclude other possible local and systemic causes of pruritus.[2–5]

Prevalence and clinical manifestations

In their original description of uraemic pruritus, Chargin and Keil reported that about 15% of patients with chronic renal insufficiency experienced pruritus.[1] However, a dramatic increase in the incidence of uraemic pruritus occurred in the 1960s, when haemodialysis treatment of chronic renal failure was introduced. Two potential explanations were suggested for this phenomenon: one was a direct role of artificial membranes in inducing pruritus; the other was the prolongation of patients' life by haemodialysis, allowing more time for pruritus to occur. More recent data suggest that as many as 30% of patients with end-stage renal failure, not requiring dialysis, experience pruritus. The prevalence of pruritus in patients on dialysis varies in different studies and centres. The highest prevalence is more than 85%.[6–12] However, some recent data indicate that the incidence of pruritus in haemodialysis patients has become less during the last decade.[11–13]

The incidence of uraemic pruritus is similar in patients on haemodialysis and on continuous ambulatory peritoneal dialysis (CAPD).[14] Psychological factors may be important as patients in self-care centres complain of pruritus less commonly.[15] The incidence of pruritus does not appear to depend on age, gender, type of dialysate, or specific underlying renal disease. No relationship has been noted between pruritus and results of routine biochemical tests (e.g. blood urea nitrogen, creatinine, uric acid, and alkaline phosphatase).[11, 16] The duration of the haemodialysis period may influence the incidence of uraemic pruritus; patients in whom haemodialysis has been discontinued experience pruritus more frequently.[11] Further, there is a positive correlation between the intensity of pruritus (total score of pruritus as well as elements of itch intensity scoring, such as: severity and sleep disturbance) and the duration of the haemodialysis period.[13] The influence of the type of dialysis membrane on the prevalence of pruritus is not clear and needs further detailed evaluation.[11] Some have found pruritus to be more common in patients undergoing haemodialysis with less biocompatible and less permeable cuprophane membranes.[10] However, these observations have been disputed.[13]

Clinical presentation

About 20–40% of uraemic patients have continuous itch with frequent exacerbations associated with dialysis sessions.[2, 11] A further 25% of patients experience pruritus only during haemodialysis.[11, 13] Pruritus may be worse in the summer, possibly due to a decrease in the threshold for the perception of pruritus due to increased skin temperature.[2, 8, 17]

Up to 20–50% of patients experience generalized pruritus.[11, 13] Although there are no preferential sites for uraemic pruritus, several authors have reported that pruritus is more common in the back (especially in patients lying down during dialysis sessions) and on the forearm with the arteriovenous shunt. The latter association may relate to frequent exposure of this area to disinfectants and other materials.[2, 11, 13]

Pathogenesis

Although uraemic pruritus was first reported 70 years ago, the pathogenesis of uraemic pruritus is still not completely clear. It is definitely multifactorial (Table 6.1).[3–5] Recently, special attention has been paid to the role of xerosis, mast cells, and neurogenic abnormalities.

Dry skin (xerosis)

Dry skin is present in most uraemic patients. In some series it has been reported in more than 80% of haemodialysis patients.[7, 8, 10, 18] Histological examination of normal-looking uraemic skin demonstrates

Table 6.1 Factors possibly involved in the pathogenesis of uraemic pruritus

Dry skin (xerosis)

Mast cell accumulation and degranulation

Decreased chymase activity

Histamine

Serotonin

Secondary hyperparathyroidism

Divalent ions

Cytokines

Bile acids

Opioid system

Cutaneous neuropathy

micro-angiopathy and atrophy of the epidermis, sebaceous glands, and the ductal portion of eccrine sweat glands.[7, 9, 19, 20] There is also impairment of sweat secretion[21] and hydration of the stratum corneum.[22] A correlation between the severity of xerosis and pruritus has been confirmed,[6, 13, 18, 22, 23] although some objective methods have failed to show a direct relationship between skin hydration and pruritus.[10, 24] The discrepancies could be attributable to different methodologies employed in the different studies. For example, the corneometer (which measures the thickness of the stratum corneum) records both the deeper and more superficial layers of the epidermis.[18] The observation that only patients with severe xerosis have continuous pruritus and the efficacy of emollients in reducing its intensity[3] also support dry skin as an important factor in uraemic pruritus.

Mast cells

In uraemic subjects mast cell production and accumulation in various organs is probably stimulated by increased concentrations of parathyroid hormone (PTH), i.e. secondary hyperparathyroidism. In contrast to the intact mast cells found in the normal upper dermis, mast cells in uraemic patients are more numerous,[9, 11, 14, 25] they are diffusely spread throughout the whole dermis, and most are degranulated.[11, 25] However, degranulation of mast cells might simply be the result of intensive scratching. Despite the above-mentioned histological changes, only a few investigators have been able to find a relationship between mast cells and pruritus.[26, 27]

Tryptase and chymase activity

Altered tryptase and chymase activity associated with reduced numbers of tryptase-positive and chymase-positive mast cells in the skin of pruritic uraemic patients may be implicated in the pathogenesis of uraemic pruritus.[11, 25] Chymase is known to degrade substance P, which directly releases histamine from mast cells, and leads hence to the development of pruritus.[28]

Histamine

Histamine is the main mediator of pruritus in several acute dermatoses. Histamine concentrations were found to be increased in plasma of patients with chronic renal insufficiency, probably due to renal retention of histamine in advanced uraemia.[29] Elevated plasma histamine levels have been reported in patients with severe uraemic pruritus,[2, 29, 30] and there may be increased sensitivity to histamine in uraemic patients.[31] Despite a smaller flare reaction to histamine in uraemia, the perception of pruritus persists and may even be augmented. However, most authors have been unable to demonstrate a significant relationship between plasma concentration of histamine and the intensity of uraemic itch.[14, 29, 32, 33] As H_1-antihistamines do not cause significant relief of uraemic pruritus,[3] histamine alone is not a major causal factor in uraemic pruritus.

Serotonin

Serotonin (5-hydroxytryptamine, 5-HT) causes pruritus peripherally through the release of histamine from cutaneous mast cells or centrally, possibly by an interaction with the opioid neurotransmitter system.[30, 34, 35] However, although serotonin blood levels are elevated in patients on haemodialysis or CAPD, they do not correlate with the intensity of pruritus.[30, 36] Clinical trials of the efficacy of ondansetron, an antagonist of 5-HT_3 receptors, yielded conflicting results.[30, 37] It is possible that the effect of ondansetron may depend on the number of cutaneous mast cells.[35] The possible role of serotonin in the pathogenesis of uraemic pruritus requires further elucidation.

Secondary hyperparathyroidism

Secondary hyperparathyroidism is a frequent complication seen in patients with advanced renal insufficiency and pruritus.[38, 39] Arguments for and against a role of PTH in the pathogenesis of uraemic pruritus are presented in Table 6.2.

Table 6.2 Arguments in favour of and against a role of parathormone (PTH) in the pathogenesis of uraemic pruritus

Evidence in favour	Evidence against
Elevated PTH is frequently associated with pruritus[58]	No pruritus in patients with high plasma PTH levels[14]
Increased plasma PTH level in pruritic patients[83]	Severe pruritus in patients with low plasma PTH levels[83]
Positive correlation between plasma PTH level and pruritus intensity[58]	No correlation between PTH and pruritus in the majority of studies[9, 38, 39]
Relationship between mid-region PTH (not intact) and pruritus[40]	Recurrence after parathyroidectomy[33]
Relief after hyperpara-thyroidectomy[33, 42]	No pruritus after intradermal injection of PTH[22]

Although PTH alone probably does not play a significant role in the pathogenesis of uraemic pruritus, mid-region PTH (m-PTH) could be a marker for other pruritogenic middle molecular weight substances, the plasma concentrations of which might be elevated in uraemic subjects with pruritus.[5]

Divalent ions

Calcium may contribute to the development of pruritus by influencing degranulation of mast cells.[40] On the other hand, increased serum concentrations of calcium and phosphate may lead to metastatic cutaneous calcification. Cutaneous calcifications are common in uraemic patients, and may stimulate itch receptors in the skin.[5, 11] Magnesium has been postulated to be involved in the neurogenic stimulation of the release of histamine from cutaneous mast cells.[41] Elevated plasma and/or skin concentrations of calcium, phosphate, magnesium, and aluminum have been demonstrated by several authors in uraemic patients. However, only a few studies have documented a significant correlation between plasma or skin divalent ion concentrations and pruritus.[6, 11, 22, 42–44]

Cytokines

Various cytokines can contribute to the development of pruritus. For example interleukin IL-2 used as a therapeutic agent for cancer patients induced pruritus,[45] and the intradermal injection of IL-2 causes severe pruritus.[46] Although IL-1 is not itself pruritogenic, it has been suggested that it causes the release of pruritogens.[2] During haemodialysis several cytokines are released due to contact of blood with dialysis membranes.[47] In addition, unidentified pruritogenic cytokines may be produced by various activated cells, when such cells accumulate in the upper dermis close to pruritus receptors. Significantly increased numbers of CD1-positive cells were found in the skin of uraemic patients with pruritus, suggesting that CD1-positive cells could be involved in the release of pruritogenic substances.[48]

Bile acids

Patients with advanced chronic renal insufficiency were found to have elevated serum levels of total bile acids. Patients with pruritus had higher levels of total bile acids than non-pruritic subjects, and a positive correlation between bile acid concentrations and the intensity of pruritus was found.[5] A role of bile acids in pathogenesis of uraemic pruritus seems to be supported by relief of uraemic pruritus by colestyramine.[49] However, colestyramine adsorbs many substances other than bile acids and some of these other substances may be pruritogenic.

Opioid system

Recently published data suggest that the increased opioidergic tone may be involved in uraemic pruritus. It has been proposed that μ-opioid receptors are pruritus-inducing, but that κ-opioid receptors are pruritus-suppressive.[5, 50] It is known that μ-opioid receptor agonists, for example, morphine, may induce pruritus and that opioid receptor antagonists, for example, naltrexone, may suppress pruritus in certain circumstances, including uraemic pruritus.

In haemodialysis patients with pruritus, expression of all opioid receptors on peripheral lymphocytes has been found to be lower than in healthy individuals. In uraemic patients with intense itching, the reduction of μ-opioid receptors was less than that for κ-opioid receptors. It was suggested that an imbalance in the expression of μ-opioid and κ-opioid receptors may contribute to the pathogenesis of uraemic pruritus.[5, 50] Moreover, a κ-opioid receptor agonist (TRK-820) significantly reduced pruritus in a mouse model,[51] and initial experience in using this agent to treat uraemic itch has been promising (Szepietowski J., unpublished data).

Skin innervation

Nerve fibres sprouting throughout the layers of the epidermis in uraemic patients have been proposed to be the morphological basis of uraemic pruritus.[2, 52] However, such morphological observations were not confirmed by other investigators.[53, 54] Most pruritic patients on haemodialysis have histological evidence of peripheral neuropathy.[55] Direct evidence for a role of neuropathy in uraemic pruritus may be relief of itching following topical application of capsaicin, an agent that induces degradation of substance P in the cutaneous nerve endings[56] and loss of sensory cutaneous fibres.[57]

Treatment

The first step should be to apply emollients regularly, once or twice daily. There is no rational basis for the use of H_1-antihistamines in uraemic pruritus.[4, 5] Selected treatment modalities that seem to be the most promising and well-documented are described below.

Enhance dialysis regimen and improve nutritional state

Patients without pruritus appear to be better dialysed and have a better nutritional state.[23] It has been postulated that higher dialysis efficacy and good nutritional status reduce the prevalence and degree of uraemic pruritus.[58] Some authors have reported a decrease of pruritus associated with the use of more permeable dialysis membranes.[48, 58, 59] A low dialysate calcium concentration may be effective in suppressing intractable uraemic pruritus. Haemodialysis with a dialysate calcium concentration of less then 1.25 mmol/l was recently advocated for short-term therapy. Patients dialysed with a low calcium concentration dialysate had substantial relief from itching. However, long-term use of such low calcium concentrations in the dialysate may lead to aggravation of renal osteodystrophy.[60]

Ultraviolet light

Ultraviolet B (UVB) therapy is now emerging as a key treatment modality. It exerts several immunomodulatory effects on human skin, and these effects are probably the most important factor underlying its effectiveness. Three main mechanisms to explain the photo-immunological effects of UV irradiation have been proposed:

- a direct effect of UVB on the synthesis of soluble mediators;

- modulation of the expression of cell-surface associated molecules;
- stimulation of cell apoptosis.[47, 61]

Several studies have confirmed the efficacy of UVB in uraemic pruritus.[62–64] Treatment seems to be well tolerated and patients usually experience longlasting remissions (mean: 18 months). The mechanism by which UVB reduces uraemic pruritus is still unclear. Several theories have been proposed. For example:

- reduction of the skin content of phosphorus, which may inhibit microprecipitation of calcium and magnesium phosphates;[63]
- reduction of vitamin A content of the skin;[62]
- suppression of histamine release from cutaneous mast cells;[65]
- alterations of cutaneous nerves;[66]
- inactivation of the unidentified circulatory pruritogens;[67]
- systemic effects, based on observations that patients receiving UVB treatment to only half of the body experience whole-body relief of pruritus;[68]
- mast cell apoptosis.[64]

A new UVB option—narrow-band UVB therapy—also seems promising. Narrow-band UVB radiation is able to penetrate further than broadband UVB into the dermis, reaching dermal-infiltrating cells, including mast cells.[61] Although preliminary experience suggests a beneficial effect of narrow-band UVB in the treatment of uraemic pruritus (Szepietowski J.C., unpublished data), controlled trials are required to determine its efficacy.

Ultraviolet A (UVA) is not effective.[70–72] Only one study has suggested a beneficial effect of topical psoralens plus UVA (PUVA)-therapy.[73]

Topical capsaicin

Capsaicin is an alkaloid isolated from the pepper of the genus *Capsicum*. It depletes substance P from nociceptor nerve endings and causes atrophy of cutaneous C fibres. Capsaicin is applied as a 0.025% or 0.075% cream 3–5 times daily. At the beginning of treatment a local burning sensation often occurs. Several studies, included placebo-controlled ones, have shown capsaicin to be effective in uraemic pruritus.[39, 56, 74] It is especially helpful when uraemic pruritus is localized. For practical reasons application of capsaicin to the whole body surface is not recommended.

Colestyramine

It has recently been suggested that bile acids may be involved in the pathogenesis of uraemic pruritus;[5, 75] if so, colestyramine may be effective. Colestyramine has been successfully used to reduce pruritus associated with intrahepatic cholestasis.[76] In uraemic patients relief of pruritus after a course of colestyramine has been reported.[49] However, this study involved only 5 patients treated with colestyramine and 5 treated with placebo.

Thalidomide

A double-blind, cross-over study of low doses of thalidomide administered at bedtime for 7 consecutive days yielded promising results. More than 50% of the patients reported improvement of their pruritus, which had been unresponsive to conventional therapy.[77] Based on this one study, which involved only 18 patients, thalidomide seems to be promising in the treatment of uraemic pruritus. However, its limited availability and adverse events profile may be problematic.

Opioid receptor antagonists and agonists

The functional status of the opioid system seems to be enhanced in patients with uraemic pruritus. Both naloxone and naltrexone, opioid receptor antagonists, have been shown to reduce severe uraemic pruritus.[78, 79] Some authors recommend an opioid receptor antagonist for persistent uraemic pruritus.[80] However, the latest randomized controlled study suggested that naltrexone is ineffective when the pruritus is only moderately severe.[12]

Serotonin type-3 receptor antagonists

In an open-label study, ondansetron, a specific 5-HT$_3$ receptor antagonist, 4 mg orally b.d., controlled uraemic pruritus in each of 11 subjects, within 2 weeks of starting treatment.[30] Relief was accompanied by a marked decrease in plasma histamine and serotonin concentrations. However, in a subsequent randomized placebo-controlled trial, ondansetron 8 mg three times daily for 1 week was not more efficacious than placebo.[37] Similar results have been obtained in a trial of ondansetron for the pruritus of cholestasis.[81] The only type of pruritus for which ondansetron is currently recommended is that induced by opioids.[82]

Conclusions

- The pathogenesis of pruritus in chronic renal insufficiency with and without dialysis treatment is complex. Multiple factors have been identified, and it is probable that most or all of them may contribute to this form of pruritus simultaneously.

- That multiple factors precipitate pruritus in patients with renal failure is reflected in the multiplicity of therapies that are used. There is no standard treatment for pruritus in uraemic patients at present.

- Treatment of dry skin (xerosis) with emollients is always important.

- Treatment with UVB phototherapy is promising and not toxic to uraemic patients.

- For localized pruritus capsaicin provides most relief.

- For severe generalized pruritus thalidomide may be the best choice.

- When pruritus is refractory, combining two or more therapies may be important.

Acknowledgements

This chapter was prepared on the basis of available data in the literature as well as our own studies. The valuable contributions of the following co-investigators is acknowledged: Tomasz Szepietowski (Wroclaw, Poland), Willem A van Vloten, Theo Thepen (Utrecht, The Netherlands), Robert A Schwartz, Arunas Urbonas (New Jersey, USA), and Akimichi Morita (Nagoya, Japan).

References

1. Chargin L, Keil H. (1932). Skin diseases in non-surgical renal disease. *Arch Dermatol Syphilol* **26**:314–35.

2. Stahle-Backdahl M. (1989). Uremic pruritus. Clinical and experimental studies. *Acta Derm Venereol Suppl (Stockh)* **145**:1–38.

3. Ponticelli C, Bencini PL. (1992). Uremic pruritus: a review. *Nephron* **60**:1–5.

4. Szepietowski JC, Schwartz RA. (1998). Uremic pruritus. *Int J Dermatol* **37**: 247–53.

5. Urbonas A, Schwartz RA, Szepietowski JC. (2001). Uremic pruritus—an update. *Am J Nephrol* **21**:343–50.

6. Young AW Jr, Sweeney EW, David DS, *et al.* (1973). Dermatologic evaluation of pruritus in patients on hemodialysis. *NY State J Med* **73**:2670–4.

7. Gilchrest BA, Rowe JW, Mihm MC Jr. (1980). Clinical and histological skin changes in chronic renal failure: evidence for a dialysis-resistant, transplant-responsive microangiopathy. *Lancet* **2**:1271–5.

8. Gilchrest BA, Stern RS, Steinman TI, Brown RS, Arndt KA, Anderson WW. (1982). Clinical features of pruritus among patients undergoing maintenance hemodialysis. *Arch Dermatol* **118**:154–6.

9. Matsumoto M, Ichimaru K, Horie A. (1985). Pruritus and mast cell proliferation of the skin in end stage renal failure. *Clin Nephrol* **23**:285–8.

10. Stahle-Backdahl M, Hägermark O, Lins LE. (1988). Pruritus in patients on maintenance hemodialysis. *Acta Med Scand* **224**:55–60.

11. Szepietowski J. (1996). Selected element of the pathogenesis of pruritus in haemodialysis patients. *Med Sci Monit* **2**:343–7.

12. Pauli-Magnus C, Mikus G, Alscher DM, *et al.* (2000). Naltrexone does not relieve uremic pruritus: results of a randomized, double-blind, placebo-controlled crossover study. *J Am Soc Nephrol* **11**:514–9.

13. Szepietowski JC, Sikora M, Kusztal M, Salomon J, Magott M, Szepietowski T. (2002). Uremic pruritus: a clinical study of maintenance hemodialysis patients. *J Dermatol* **29**:621–7.

14. Mettang T, Fritz P, Weber J, Machleidt C, Hubel E, Kuhlmann U. (1990). Uremic pruritus in patients on hemodialysis or continuous ambulatory peritoneal dialysis (CAPD). The role of plasma histamine and skin mast cells. *Clin Nephrol* **34**:136–41.

15. Tapia L. (1979). Pruritus on hemodialysis. *Int J Dermatol* **18**:217–18.

16. Jakic M. (1999). Does uremic pruritus in hemodialyzed patients disappear only with replacement therapy? *Lijec Vjesn* **121**:118–22.

17. Francos GC. (1997). Uremic pruritus. *Semin Dial* **75**:48–53.

18. Triebskorn A, Gloor M, Greiner F. (1983). Comparative investigations on the water content of the stratum corneum using different methods of measurement. *Dermatologica* **167**:64–9.

19. Rosenthal SR. (1931). Uremic dermatitis. *Arch Dermatol Syph* **23**:934–45.

20. Landing BH, Wells TR, Williamson ML. (1970). Anatomy of eccrine sweat glands in children with chronic renal insufficiency and other fatal chronic diseases. *Am J Clin Pathol* **54**:15–21.

21. Rosen T. (1979). Uremic pruritus: a review. *Cutis* **23**:790–2.

22. Morton CA, Lafferty M, Hau C, Henderson I, Jones M, Lowe JG. (1996). Pruritus and skin hydration during dialysis. *Nephrol Dial Transplant* **11**:2031–6.

23. Goicoechea M, de Sequera P, Ochando A, Andrea C, Caramelo C. (1999). Uremic pruritus: an unresolved problem in hemodialysis patients. *Nephron* **82**:73–4.

24. Yosipovitch G, Tur E, Morduchowicz G, Boner G. (1993). Skin surface pH, moisture, and pruritus in haemodialysis patients. *Nephrol Dial Transplant* **8**:1129–32.

25. Szepietowski J, Thepen T, van Vloten WA, Szepietowski T, Bihari IC. (1995). Pruritus and mast cell proliferation in the skin of haemodialysis patients. *Inflamm Res* **44** (Suppl. 1):S84–5.

26. Dimkovic N, Djukanovic L, Radmilovic A, Bojic P, Juloski T. (1992). Uremic pruritus and skin mast cells. *Nephron* **61**:5–9.

27. Leong SO, Tan CC, Lye WC, Lee EJ, Chan HL. (1994). Dermal mast cell density and pruritus in end-stage renal failure. *Ann Acad Med Singapore* **23**:327–9.

28. Greaves MW, Wall PD. (1996). Pathophysiology of itching. *Lancet* **348**:938–40.

29. Stockenhuber F, Kurz RW, Sertl K, Grimm G, Balcke P. (1990). Increased plasma histamine levels in uraemic pruritus. *Clin Sci (Lond)* **79**:477–82.

30. Balaskas EV, Bamihas GI, Karamouzis M, Voyiatzis G, Tourkantonis A. (1998). Histamine and serotonin in uremic pruritus: effect of ondansetron in CAPD-pruritic patients. *Nephron* **78**:395–402.

31. Stahle-Backdahl M. (1988). Stratum corneum hydration in patients undergoing maintenance hemodialysis. *Acta Derm Venereol* **68**:531–4.

32. Piazza V, De Filippi C, Aprile C, *et al.* (1993). Uraemic pruritus and plasma histamine concentrations. *Nephrol Dial Transplant* **8**:670–1.

33. Matsui C, Ida M, Hamada M, Morohashi M, Hasegawa M. (1994). Effects of azelastin on pruritus and plasma histamine levels in hemodialysis patients. *Int J Dermatol* **33**:868–71.

34. Hägermark O. (1992). Peripheral and central mediators of itch. *Skin Pharmacol* **5**:1–8.

35. Weisshaar E, Ziethen B, Rohl FW, Gollnick H. (1999). The antipruritic effect of a 5-HT$_3$ receptor antagonist (tropisetron) is dependent on mast cell depletion—an experimental study. *Exp Dermatol* **8**:254–60.

36. Kerr PG, Argiles A, Mion C. (1992). Whole blood serotonin levels are markedly elevated in patients on dialytic therapy. *Am J Nephrol* **12**:14–8.

37. Ashmore SD, Jones CH, Newstead CG, Daly MJ, Chrystyn H. (2000). Ondansetron therapy for uremic pruritus in hemodialysis patients. *Am J Kidney Dis* **35**:827–31.

38. Massry SG, Popovtzer MM, Coburn JW, Makoff DL, Maxwell MH, Kleeman CR. (1968). Intractable pruritus as a manifestation of secondary hyper-parathyroidism in uremia. Disappearance of itching after subtotal parathyroidectomy. *N Engl J Med* **279**:697–700.

39. Cho YL, Liu HN, Huang TP, Tarng DC. (1997). Uremic pruritus: roles of parathyroid hormone and substance P. *J Am Acad Dermatol* **36**:538–43.

40. Ahmad S. (1993). Uremic pruritus. *Semin Dial* **6**:348–50.

41. Graf H, Kovarik J, Stummvoll HK, Wolf A. (1979). Disappearance of uraemic pruritus after lowering dialysate magnesium concentration. *Br Med J* **2**:1478–9.

42. Carmichael AJ, Dickinson F, McHugh MI, Martin AM, Farrow M. (1988). Magnesium free dialysis for uraemic pruritus. *Br Med J* **297**:1584–5.

43. Ostlere LS, Taylor C, Baillod R, Wright S. (1994). Relationship between pruritus, transepidermal water loss, and biochemical markers of renal itch in haemodialysis patients. *Nephrol Dial Transplant* **9**:1302–4.

44. Friga V, Linos A, Linos DA. (1997). Is aluminum toxicity responsible for uremic pruritus in chronic hemodialysis patients? *Nephron* **75**:48–53.

45. Gaspari AA, Lotze MT, Rosenberg SA, Stern JB, Katz SI. (1987). Dermatologic changes associated with interleukin 2 administration. *JAMA* **258**:1624–9.

46. Wahlgren CF, Tengvall Linder M, Hägermark O, Scheynius A. (1995). Itch and inflammation induced by intradermally injected interleukin-2 in atopic dermatitis patients and healthy subjects. *Arch Dermatol Res* **287**:572–80.

47. Pereira BJ, Dinarello CA. (1994). Production of cytokines and cytokine inhibitory proteins in patients on dialysis. *Nephrol Dial Transplant* **9** (Suppl. 2):60–71.

48. Szepietowski J, Thepen T, Szepietowski T. (1996). Phenotype analysis of cell infiltrate in normal-looking skin of hemodialysis patients. *Acta Dermatovenerol Croat* **4**:3–6.

49. Silverberg DS, Iaina A, Reisin E, Rotzak R, Eliahou HE. (1977). Cholestyramine in uraemic pruritus. *Br Med J* **1**:752–3.

50. Odou P, Azar R, Luyckx M, Brunet C, Dine T. (2001). A hypothesis for endogenous opioid peptides in uraemic pruritus: role of enkephalin. *Nephrol Dial Transplant* **16**:1953–4.

51. Togashi Y, Umeuchi H, Okano K, *et al.* (2002). Antipruritic activity of the kappa-opioid receptor agonist, TRK-820. *Eur J Pharmacol* **435**:259–64.

52. Johansson O, Hilliges M, Stahle-Backdahl M. (1989). Intraepidermal neuron-specific enolase (NSE)-immunoreactive nerve fibres: evidence for sprouting in uremic patients on maintenance hemodialysis. *Neurosci Lett* **99**:281–6.

53. Fantini F, Baraldi A, Pincelli A. (1990). Neuron-specific enolase-immunoreactive fibres in uremic patients. *Acta Derm Venereol* **70**:363–5.

54. Szepietowski J, Thepen T, van Vloten WA, Szepietowski T. (1993). Tyrosine hydroxylase immunoreactive fibres in the skin of hemodialysed patients. *Acta Derm Venerol (Stockh)* **74**:75.

55. Jedras M, Zakrzewska-Pniewska B, Wardyn K, Switalski M. (1998). Uremic neuropathy—II. Is pruritus in dialyzed patients related to neuropathy? *Pol Arch Med Wewn* **99**:462–9.

56. Breneman DL, Cardone JS, Blumsack RF, Lather RM, Searle EA, Pollack VE. (1992). Topical capsaicin for treatment of hemodialysis-related pruritus. *J Am Acad Dermatol* **26**:91–4.

57. Lynn B. (1992). Capsaicin: actions on C fibre afferents that may be involved in itch. *Skin Pharmacol* **5**:9–13.

58. Hiroshige K, Kabashima N, Takasugi M, Kuroiwa A. (1995). Optimal dialysis improves uremic pruritus. *Am J Kidney Dis* **25**:413–9.

59. Robertson KE, Mueller BA. (1996). Uremic pruritus. *Am J Health Syst Pharm* **53**:2159–70.

60. Kyriazis J, Glotsos J. (2000). Dialysate calcium concentration of ≤ 1.25 mmol/l: is it effective in suppressing uremic pruritus? *Nephron* **84**:85–6.

61. Krutmann J, Morita A. (1999). Mechanisms of ultraviolet UVB and UVA phototherapy. *J Invest Dermatol Symp Proc* **4**:70–2.

62. Berne B, Vahlquist A, Fischer T, Danielson BG, Berne C. (1984). UV treatment of uraemic pruritus reduces the vitamin A content of the skin. *Eur J Clin Invest* **14**:203–6.

63. Blachley JD, Blankenship DM, Menter A, Parker TF 3rd, Knochel JP. (1985). Uremic pruritus: skin divalent ion content and response to ultraviolet phototherapy. *Am J Kidney Dis* **5**:237–41.

64. Szepietowski JC, Morita A, Tsuji T. (2002). Ultraviolet B induces mast cell apoptosis: a hypothetical mechanism of ultraviolet B treatment for uraemic pruritus. *Med Hypotheses* **58**:167–70.

65. Imazu LE, Tachibana T, Danno K, Tanaka M, Imamura S. (1993). Histamine-releasing factor(s) in sera of uraemic pruritus patients in a possible mechanism of UVB therapy. *Arch Dermatol Res* **285**:423–7.

66. Kumakiri M, Hashimoto K, Willis I. (1978). Biological changes of human cutaneous nerves caused by ultraviolet irradiation: an ultrastructural study. *Br J Dermatol* **99**:65–75.

67. Schultz BC, Roenigk HH Jr. (1980). Uremic pruritus treated with ultraviolet light. *J Am Med Assoc* **243**:1836–7.

68. Gilchrest BA. (1979). Ultraviolet phototherapy of uremic pruritus. *Int J Dermatol* **18**:741–8.

69. Gilchrest BA, Rowe JW, Brown RS, Steinman TI, Arndt KA. (1979). Ultraviolet phototherapy of uremic pruritus. Long-term results and possible mechanism of action. *Ann Intern Med* **91**:17–21.

70. Hindson C, Taylor A, Martin A, Downey A. (1981). UVA light for relief of uraemic pruritus. *Lancet* **1**:215.

71. Taylor R, Taylor AE, Diffey BL, Hindson TC. (1983). A placebo-controlled trial of UV-A phototherapy for the treatment of uraemic pruritus. *Nephron* **33**:14–16.

72. Henry A, Tetzlaff JE, Steckner K. (2002). Ondansetron is effective in treatment of pruritus after intrathecal fentanyl. *Reg Anesth Pain Med* **27**:538–40.

73. Uesugi Y, Kamasaka N, Okada Y, Ito S, Matsumara N, Tagami H. (1996). Topical chemotherapy (PUVA) for the relief of uremic pruritus in patients undergoing hemodialysis. *J Dermatol Ther* **7**:247–9.

74. Tarng DC, Cho YL, Liu HN, Huang TP. (1996). Hemodialysis-related pruritus: a double-blind, placebo-controlled, crossover study of capsaicin 0.025% cream. *Nephron* **72**:617–22.

75. Quist RG, Ton-Nu HT, Lillienau J, Hofmann AF, Barrett KE. (1991). Activation of mast cells by bile acids. *Gastroenterology* **101**:446–56.

76. Datta DV, Sherlock S. (1966). Cholestyramine for long term relief of the pruritus complicating intrahepatic cholestasis. *Gastroenterology* **50**:323–32.

77. Silva SR, Viana PC, Lugon NV, Hoette M, Ruzany F, Lugon JR. (1994). Thalidomide for the treatment of uremic pruritus: a crossover randomized double-blind trial. *Nephron* **67**:270–3.

78. Andersen LW, Friedberg M, Lokkegaard N. (1984). Naloxone in the treatment of uremic pruritus: a case history. *Clin Nephrol* **21**:355–6.

79. Peer G, Kivity S, Agami O, *et al.* (1996). Randomised crossover trial of naltrexone in uraemic pruritus. *Lancet* **348**:1552–4.

80. Schwartz IF, Iaina A. (1999). Uraemic pruritus. *Nephrol Dial Transplant* **14**: 834–9.

81. O'Donohue JW, Haigh C, Williams R. (1997). Ondansetron in the treatment of pruritus of cholestasis: a randomised controlled trial. *Gastroenterology* **112**:A1349.

82. Twycross R, Greaves MW, Handwerker H, *et al.* (2003). Itch: scratching more than the surface. *QJM* **96**:7–26.

83. Carmichael AJ, McHugh MM, Martin AM, Farrow M. (1988). Serological markers of renal itch in patients receiving long term haemodialysis. *Br Med J* (*Clin Res Ed*) **296**:1575.

7

Opioid-induced pruritus

Małgorzata Krajnik

The magnitude of the problem

Pruritus is a common adverse effect of spinal opioid administration, occurring in up to 90% of patients.[1, 2] However, the incidence of pruritus after systemic administration is probably not higher then 1%.[1] Obstetric patients seem to be more susceptible to opioid-induced pruritus, probably due to interaction with oestrogens.[3, 4] There are also differences among opioids: morphine and sufentanil are more pruritogenic than fentanyl and butorphanol.[5-7] Although intradermally injected morphine and methadone (and some other opioids) achieve a very high local opioid tissue concentration, release histamine from mast cells, and cause localized pruritus, this is *not* comparable to the more generalized pruritus seen after clinical doses of opioids (see Chapter 2).[8, 9]

Pathogenesis of pruritus induced by spinal opioids

Pruritus usually occurs within 6–12 hours after intrathecal administration.[10] This suggests that the drug needs to be transported first cephalad. Pruritus is more common when spinal opioids are given intrathecally rather than epidurally[11] and becomes less common with subsequent doses.[12] The rapid development of tolerance may be the reason why patients treated for cancer pain with spinal opioids for weeks or months do not suffer from pruritus after the first or second day.[13] Localization of pruritus may vary with opioid used. In one study, epidural fentanyl was associated with segmental pruritus, whereas epidural morphine caused generalized pruritus.[14]

Although pruritus has been associated with all opioids given spinally, concurrent drug administration may alter the incidence. For example, there is a higher frequency and intensity of pruritus with fentanyl when it is combined with intrathecal procaine compared with lidocaine.[15] In a systematic review of 22 randomized controlled trials of spinal opioids, about 60% of patients receiving an opioid without an antipruritic drug had some pruritus.[15, 16]

It has been suggested that pruritus induced by spinal opioids is mediated by μ-opioid receptors. This hypothesis is supported by two indirect observations: (1) κ-opioid receptor agonists are antipruritic; (2) naloxone, which is a non-selective antagonist of all opioid receptors, relieves opioid-induced pruritus.[16]

Pruritus due to spinal opioids is usually limited to the face, neck, and/or upper thorax, especially in the facial area innervated by the trigeminal nerve. The spinal nucleus of the trigeminal nerve is rich in opioid receptors. At the level of the third or fourth cervical segment of the cord, the spinal nucleus and tract of trigeminal nerve have continuity with the substantia gelatinosa. Therefore, cells in the grey matter of the dorsal horn have indirect access to trigeminal nuclei by spino-trigeminal interneurons that travel in the anterolateral quadrant of the cord.[17] This is the rationale behind the suggestion that there is a multisynaptic pruritus reflex from the substantia gelatinosa to the nucleus of the trigeminal nerve in the medulla.[18] The reflex might be relayed at the central level by a medullary pruritus centre.

Animal studies suggested that this pruritus centre lies in the caudal part of the floor of the fourth cerebral ventricle and is functionally linked to the trigeminal nucleus involved in the pruritus reflex.[2, 19] In man, itching localized to the nostrils is seen in association with tumour infiltrating the floor of the fourth ventricle.[20] With spinal opioids a segmental distribution of itching spreading rostrally from the site of injection is frequently observed, suggesting that it is probably due to cephalad spread of the opioids in the cerebrospinal fluid and interaction with the trigeminal nucleus and nerve roots.[1] Studies with monkeys in which different opioids were injected into the medullary dorsal horn support the view that the medullary dorsal horn is a site where μ-opioid receptor agonists act to produce facial-scratching behaviour.[18, 21] Thus, opioid-induced pruritus is probably neurogenic in origin, resulting from a spinal reflex transmitted through a medullary pruritus centre associated with the spinal nucleus of the trigeminal nerve.[17, 18] This transmission may be blocked by small amount of local anaesthetic added to the spinal opioid.[17] Morphine injected intracisternally to mice increased facial pruritus, but the same or a higher dose of morphine given intradermally did not produce the same effect.[21] These observations support a central origin for pruritus following central administration of opioids. Both naltrexone (an opioid receptor antagonist) and cetirizine, an H_1-antihistamine, significantly diminished histamine-induced itching in a human study.[22] Cetirizine reduced the vascular reaction to histamine, a peripheral effect, whereas naltrexone diminished alloknesis, a central effect. This further supported evidence of centrally mediated opioid-induced pruritus. Apart from stimulation of a pruritus centre and spinal trigeminal nuclei, morphine may have an excitatory effect on central ascending neuronal tracts resulting in pruritus secondary to activation of serotoninergic pathways. It is suggested from animal studies that morphine may produce part of its analgesic effect through serotonin release.[23] Thus, the inhibition of serotonin receptors may block neuronal activity and attenuate pruritus.[24–27] Another hypothesis about spinal opioid-induced pruritus is that opioid antagonism of the inhibitory transmitter glycine and gamma aminobutyric acid (GABA) may be responsible for the pruritus.[1]

In summary, none of the evidence contradicts the view that segmental pruritus after spinal opioids is a manifestation of local excitation by opioids within the spinal cord. This excitation may be amplified by prostaglandins. In one study diclofenac was able to attenuate pruritus induced by spinal opioids.[28]

Treatment of pruritus induced by spinal opioids

H_1-antihistamines

Opioid-induced pruritus responds readily to several different drugs (Table 7.1). In one study intramuscular promethazine 25 mg (an H_1-antihistamine) given postoperatively abolished pruritus caused by spinal opioids. However, this effect was insufficiently evaluated by the authors.[10] In another study, premedication with oral promethazine 10 mg was ineffective.[29] The weaker H_1-antihistamine, diphenhydramine 30 mg intravenously (IV), was also ineffective in the treatment of postoperative pruritus in women after Caesarean section.[30] In conclusion, the evidence for an antipruritic action of H_1-antihistamines on spinal opioid-induced pruritus is lacking.

Opioid antagonists

The most effective treatment is an opioid antagonist such as naloxone, but there is need to be careful so as not to reverse analgesia.[17] In a randomized

Table 7.1 Spinal opioid-induced pruritus: mechanisms and treatment options

Hypothetical mechanism	Treatment
H_1-antihistaminic effect	Promethazine IV,[10] not confirmed by others.
Enhancement of 5-HT transmission	5-HT$_3$-receptor antagonists (e.g. ondansetron IV).[9, 24, 30, 45, 60, 61, 71] However, not confirmed in a systematic review[16]
Decrease of local excitation	Bupivacaine spinally.[48] Propofol appeared not effective[16]
Stimulation of μ_2-opioid receptors	Butorphanol,[5] nalbuphine[16,34,35]
Decrease of excitation by prostaglandins	Diclofenac[28]

controlled trial IV infusion of low-dose naloxone decreased the incidence of opioid-related adverse effects, including pruritus, while maintaining analgesia.[31] Another controlled study demonstrated that epidural naloxone also reduces morphine-induced pruritus and nausea without affecting analgesia by epidural morphine and bupivacaine.[32] Nalbuphine, which has μ-opioid receptor partial agonist and κ-opioid receptor agonist properties, reversed opioid-induced pruritus without compromising analgesia in several studies.[33–40]

Butorphanol and other κ-agonists

In a human study, intranasal butorphanol, a strong κ-opioid receptor agonist and a weak μ-opioid receptor antagonist, reduced spinal opioid-induced pruritus without reversing the analgesic effects of opioid therapy.[41] Because it has higher affinity for the μ_2-opioid receptor than fentanyl and morphine, it may function as a competitive antagonist when given with other opioids. Probably, activation of μ_2-opioid receptors is responsible for the adverse effects of spinal opioids. Antagonism of the μ_2-opioid receptors may thus explain the antipruritic effect after intranasal butorphanol administration.

There is also another hypothesis that may explain the efficacy of butorphanol and nalbuphine in treatment of spinal opioid-induced pruritus. Both drugs are κ-opioid receptor agonists. In animal studies, a selective κ-opioid receptor agonist suppressed both antihistamine-sensitive and antihistamine-resistant pruritus via κ-opioid receptors,[42] and a selective κ-opioid receptor antagonist induced pruritus.[43, 44] Thus, there is a suggestion that κ-opioid receptor agonists may have antipruritic activity.

Serotonin antagonists

Another treatment option, without a risk of reversing analgesia, is the antagonism of 5-HT$_3$-receptors. Ondansetron, a 5-HT$_3$-receptor antagonist, relieves pruritus associated with intrathecal morphine.[24–27, 30, 37, 45, 46] A randomized controlled trial of IV ondansetron 8 mg demonstrated benefit in 70% of patients within 1 hour.[24] Because of the safety of this method, in some centres ondansetron is used as the first-line treatment of spinal opioid-induced pruritus, if the concurrent administration of a local anaesthetic does not prevent it. However, in another randomized controlled trial, prophylactic intravenous ondansetron, 8 mg, after Caesarean section under intrathecal sufentanil and morphine analgesia reduced the frequency and the severity of postoperative nausea and vomiting, but not that of pruritus.[47]

Bupivacaine

The potential of opioids to induce local excitation within the spinal cord may explain why addition of small amount of bupivacaine to the spinal opioids leads to a decrease of incidence in the segmental pruritus.[17, 48]

Propofol

One randomized controlled trial suggested that subhypnotic doses of propofol may prevent postoperative pruritus without affecting analgesia.[49–51] However, two other randomized controlled trials did not find that the antipruritic activity of propofol was greater than that of intralipid.[52–54] In yet another study nalbuphine was more efficacious in relieving pruritus than propofol.[37]

Droperidol

Whether IV droperidol is efficacious in reducing epidural morphine-induced pruritus is uncertain.[55, 56] In a recent randomized controlled trial, a postoperative epidural infusion of droperidol significantly decreased the frequency and severity of pruritus, whereas IV droperidol was ineffective.[57]

Miscellaneous

A different approach to prevent pruritus after intrathecal sufentanil is to limit the spread of the drug by adding dextrose to make a hyperbaric solution. However, although 5% dextrose added to sufentanil resulted in more localized pruritus, it also reduced the duration of analgesia.[58] In a recent randomized controlled trial, the addition of hyperbaric 3.5% dextrose to intrathecal sufentanil reduced the incidence of pruritus without affecting the duration or quality of analgesia in early labour.[59] Even if pruritus appeared, its distribution was limited to below T6 suggesting that pruritus with intrathecal sufentanil is mediated at the spinal level.

Another treatment option is to administer nonsteroidal anti-inflammatory drugs (NSAIDs) systemically. These drugs probably act by inhibiting the synthesis and release of prostaglandins in the spinal cord. In one randomized controlled trial, rectal administration of diclofenac significantly reduced the incidence and severity of postoperative morphine-induced pruritus.[28]

Treatments that appear to be promising in initial studies are often shown to lack efficacy in later studies. A recent review of randomized, controlled trials of interventions believed to be antipruritic included 1477 surgical patients. It concluded that only naloxone, naltrexone, nalbufine, and droperidol are effective in the prevention of opioid-induced pruritus. There was a lack of evidence for any antipruritic efficacy of prophylactic propofol, epidural or intrathecal epinephrine (adrenaline), epidural clonidine, epidural prednisone, intravenous ondansetron, or intramuscular hydroxyzine.[16] After publication of this analysis, other studies were published that again suggested that intravenous ondansetron may be effective in relieving spinal opioid-induced pruritus.[30, 45, 60, 61]

Pathogenesis of pruritus induced by systemic opioids

Why do systemic opioids precipitate significantly less pruritus then intrathecal opioids? If systemic opioid agonists reach the central nervous system (CNS) in a sufficient concentration to produce analgesia, then they also reach the medullary dorsal horn. So, why is opioid-induced pruritus rare after systemic administration? Based on a study with monkeys, it has been proposed that morphine has antipruritogenic activity at a non-medullary dorsal horn locus that inhibits the ability of the dorsal horn-administered morphine to induce pruritus and scratching.[62] This would explain how systemic morphine was able to inhibit the effects of morphine injected into the medullary dorsal horn. One site where morphine may act to attenuate pruritus is the midbrain. Only midbrain lesions have been found to augment scratching associated with the administration of morphine into the fourth ventricle of cats.[19] This is in agreement with the hypothesis of an opioid-agonist-activated control system of pruritus and the idea that morphine has both pruritogenic and antipruritogenic activity, depending on penetration.[62]

The mechanisms underlying pruritus caused by systemic opioids may therefore be completely different from those responsible for that caused by spinal opioids. In the case of systemic opioid administration, the itching is mostly generalized, whereas spinal opioid-induced pruritus has a clear segmental or facial distribution. Morphine induces weal and flare reactions when injected intradermally in clinically relevant doses.[63] Such reactions are presumed to result from histamine release from tissue mast cells. The development of urticaria along the vein into which morphine has been administered may be observed. Plasma concentrations of histamine may increase after IV administration of morphine but not after IV fentanyl.[63, 64] In contrast, plasma concentrations of histamine are not elevated after epidural morphine administration.[11]

The effects of different opioids have been examined *in vitro*. Histamine release induced by morphine is much greater than that induced by oxymorphone and fentanyl. Thus, histamine release does not parallel the analgesic potency of opioids.[8] The failure of naloxone to prevent histamine release from human mast cells by morphine suggests that the release process does not involve an opioid receptor.[8] Recent evidence indicates that morphine causes histamine release through opioid-receptor independent G-protein activation.[65] Cromolyn, which counteracts G-protein activation, reduced morphine-induced histamine release via opioid-independent G-protein activation.[65] Other conditions, such as preoperative medication or concurrently administered anaesthetic agent or surgical manipulation, may also exacerbate histamine release.

There are some situations in which the frequency of pruritus due to systemically administered opioids is increased. The incidence of pruritus associated with IV patient-controlled analgesia (PCA) after surgery is particularly high, for example, when PCA is used to relieve pain after Caesarean section (25% post-Caesarean section versus 5% in the general population).[66]

Treatment of pruritus induced by systemic opioids (Table 7.2)

Opioid switch

If the pruritus is a problem for the patient, it probably makes sense to change to another opioid.[67] Although opioids differ in their potential to release

Table 7.2 Treatment of pruritus induced by systemic administration of opioids

Hypothetical mechanism	Treatment
Histamine-releasing potential of different opioids varies	Opioid switch, e.g. change from morphine to hydromorphone,[67] morphine to fentanyl, or morphine to oxycodone. Probably less important than thought before. Administration of sedative H_1-antihistamines as a general measure
Opioid receptor-mediated reaction	1. Opioid switch 2. μ-opioid receptor antagonists and κ-opioid receptor agonists 3. Partial μ-opioid receptor agonists
Restoration of central inhibition and modulation of ascending pruritic impulses	Paroxetine,[70] ondansetron?[72]

histamine from the mast cells,[8] this property probably is not important here. Opioids may differ in their intrinsic activity on μ- and κ-opioid receptors. This is particularly true for butorphanol or buprenorphine.[42, 68]

Miscellaneous

Another possibility is to treat the patient with sedating H_1-antihistamines.[69] Newer, non-sedating antihistamines are not effective. When opioid rotation or H_1-antihistamines are not effective, paroxetine may be effective.[70] A recent randomized controlled trial in volunteers demonstrated an antipruritic effect of orally administered methylnaltrexone, a peripherally acting μ-opioid receptor antagonist, when this drug was given before IV morphine.[9] Thus, peripherally acting μ-opioid receptor antagonists may be promising and safe for relieving (systemic) opioid-induced pruritus.

Conclusions

• The pruritus centre is probably localized in the brainstem, but pruritus after spinal opioids is a manifestation of opioid-induced local excitation within the spinal cord.

- Pruritus due to spinal opioids is probably mediated by μ-opioid receptor agonists.
- Naloxone in small doses may attenuate pruritus without reversing analgesia.
- κ-opioid receptor agonists may have antipruritic activity.
- In some centres ondansetron is used as the treatment of choice for spinal opioid-induced pruritus.
- Opioid-induced excitation in the spinal cord can be attenuated by diclofenac, droperidol, and bupivacaine, but not by propofol.
- For pruritus induced by systemic opioids, opioid switch and oral metheylnaltrexone are advocated.

References

1. Ballantyne JC, Loach AB, Carr DB. (1988). Itching after epidural and spinal opiates. *Pain* **33**:149–60.
2. Kam PC, Tan KH. (1996). Pruritus—itching for a cause and relief? *Anaesthesia* **51**:1133–8.
3. Kelly MC, Carabine UA, Mirakhur RK. (1998). Intrathecal diamorphine for analgesia after caesarean section. A dose finding study and assessment of side-effects. *Anaesthesia* **53**:231–7.
4. Fuller JG, McMorland GH, Douglas MJ, Palmer L. (1990). Epidural morphine for analgesia after caesarean section: a report of 4880 patients. *Can J Anaesth* **37**:636–40.
5. Palacios QT, Jones MM, Hawkins JL, *et al.* (1991). Post-caesarean section analgesia: a comparison of epidural butorphanol and morphine. *Can J Anaesth* **38**:24–30.
6. Caldwell LE, Rosen MA, Shnider SM. (1994). Subarachnoid morphine and fentanyl for labor analgesia. Efficacy and adverse effects. *Reg Anesth* **19**:2–8.
7. Camann WR, Minzter BH, Denney RA, Datta S. (1993). Intrathecal sufentanil for labor analgesia. Effects of added epinephrine. *Anesthesiology* **78**:870–4.
8. Hermens JM, Ebertz JM, Hanifin JM, Hirshman CA. (1985). Comparison of histamine release in human skin mast cells induced by morphine, fentanyl, and oxymorphone. *Anesthesiology* **62**:124–9.
9. Yuan CS, Foss JF, O'Connor M, Osinski J, Roizen MF, Moss J. (1998). Efficacy of orally administered methylnaltrexone in decreasing subjective effects after intravenous morphine. *Drug Alcohol Depend* **52**:161–5.
10. Slappendel R, Weber EW, Benraad B, van Limbeek J, Dirksen R. (2000). Itching after intrathecal morphine. Incidence and treatment. *Eur J Anaesthesiol* **17**: 616–21.

11. Rawal N, Nuutinen L, Raj PP, *et al.* (1991). Behavioral and histopathologic effects following intrathecal administration of butorphanol, sufentanil, and nalbuphine in sheep. *Anesthesiology* **75**:1025–34.

12. Arner S, Rawal N, Gustafsson LL. (1988). Clinical experience of long-term treatment with epidural and intrathecal opioids—a nationwide survey. *Acta Anaesthesiol Scand* **32**:253–9.

13. Cousins MJ, Mather LE. (1984). Intrathecal and epidural administration of opioids. *Anesthesiology* **61**:276–310.

14. White MJ, Berghausen EJ, Dumont SW, *et al.* (1992). Side effects during continuous epidural infusion of morphine and fentanyl. *Can J Anaesth* **39**:576–82.

15. Mulroy MF, Larkin KL, Siddiqui A. (2001). Intrathecal fentanyl-induced pruritus is more severe in combination with procaine than with lidocaine or bupivacaine. *Reg Anesth Pain Med* **26**:252–6.

16. Kjellberg F, Tramer MR. (2001). Pharmacological control of opioid-induced pruritus: a quantitative systematic review of randomized trials. *Eur J Anaesthesiol* **18**:346–57.

17. Scott PV, Fischer HB. (1982). Intraspinal opiates and itching: a new reflex? *Br Med J (Clin Res Ed)* **284**:1015–16.

18. Thomas DA, Williams GM, Iwata K, Kenshalo DR Jr, Dubner R. (1993). The medullary dorsal horn. A site of action of morphine in producing facial scratching in monkeys. *Anesthesiology* **79**:548–54.

19. Koeningstein H. (1948). Experimental study of itch stimuli in animals. *Arch Dermatol* **57**:828–49.

20. Andreev VC, Petkov I. (1975). Skin manifestations associated with tumours of the brain. *Br J Dermatol* **92**:675–8.

21. Tohda C, Yamaguchi T, Kuraishi Y. (1997). Intracisternal injection of opioids induces itch-associated response through mu-opioid receptors in mice. *Jpn J Pharmacol* **74**:77–82.

22. Heyer G, Dotzer M, Diepgen TL, Handwerker HO. (1997). Opiate and H1 antagonist effects on histamine induced pruritus and alloknesis. *Pain* **73**: 239–43.

23. Richardson BP. (1990). Serotonin and nociception. *Ann NY Acad Sci* **600**: 511–19.

24. Borgeat A, Stirnemann HR. (1999). Ondansetron is effective to treat spinal or epidural morphine-induced pruritus. *Anesthesiology* **90**:432–6.

25. Arai L, Stayer S, Schwartz R, Dorsey A. (1996). The use of ondansetron to treat pruritus associated with intrathecal morphine in two paediatric patients. *Paediatr Anaesth* **6**:337–9.

26. Larijani GE, Goldberg ME, Rogers KH. (1996). Treatment of opioid-induced pruritus with ondansetron: report of four patients. *Pharmacotherapy* **16**: 958–60.

27. Baldo A, Sammarco E, Plaitano R, Martinelli V, Monfrecola. (2002). Narrowband (TL-01) ultraviolet B phototherapy for pruritus in polycythaemia vera. *Br J Dermatol* **147**:979–81.

28. Colbert S, O'Hanlon DM, Galvin S, Chambers F, Moriarty DC. (1999). The effect of rectal diclofenac on pruritus in patients receiving intrathecal morphine. *Anaesthesia* **54**:948–52.

29. Tarkkila P, Torn K, Tuominen M, Lindgren L. (1995). Premedication with promethazine and transdermal scopolamine reduces the incidence of nausea and vomiting after intrathecal morphine. *Acta Anaesthesiol Scand* **39**:983–6.

30. Yeh HM, Chen LK, Lin CJ, *et al.* (2000). Prophylactic intravenous ondansetron reduces the incidence of intrathecal morphine-induced pruritus in patients undergoing cesarean delivery. *Anesth Analg* **91**:172–5.

31. Gan TJ, Ginsberg B, Glass PS, Fortney J, Jhaveri R, Perno R. (1997). Opioid-sparing effects of a low-dose infusion of naloxone in patient-administered morphine sulfate. *Anesthesiology* **87**:1075–81.

32. Choi JH, Lee J, Choi JH, Bishop MJ. (2000). Epidural naloxone reduces pruritus and nausea without affecting analgesia by epidural morphine in bupivacaine. *Can J Anaesth* **47**:33–7.

33. Somrat C, Oranuch K, Ketchada U, Siriprapa S, Thipawan R. (1999). Optimal dose of nalbuphine for treatment of intrathecal-morphine induced pruritus after caesarean section. *J Obstet Gynaecol Res* **25**:209–13.

34. Cohen SE, Ratner EF, Kreitzman TR, Archer JH, Mignano LR. (1992). Nalbuphine is better than naloxone for treatment of side effects after epidural morphine. *Anesth Analg* **75**:747–52.

35. Penning JP, Samson B, Baxter AD. (1988). Reversal of epidural morphine-induced respiratory depression and pruritus with nalbuphine. *Can J Anaesth* **35**:599–604.

36. Elias M. (1997). Nalbuphine and pruritus. *Anaesthesia* **52**:613.

37. Charuluxananan S, Kyokong O, Somboonviboon W, Lertmaharit S, Ngamprasertwong P, Nimcharoendee K. (2001). Nalbuphine versus propofol for treatment of intrathecal morphine-induced pruritus after cesarean delivery. *Anesth Analg* **93**:162–5.

38. Kendrick WD, Woods AM, Daly MY, Birch RF, DiFazio C. (1996). Naloxone versus nalbuphine infusion for prophylaxis of epidural morphine-induced pruritus. *Anesth Analg* **82**:641–7.

39. Davies GG, From R. (1988). A blinded study using nalbuphine for prevention of pruritus induced by epidural fentanyl. *Anesthesiology* **69**:763–5.

40. Bruynzeel DP, de Boer EM. (1997). Waitresses' itch? *Contact Dermatitis* **36**:308.

41. Dunteman E, Karanikolas M, Filos KS. (1996). Transnasal butorphanol for the treatment of opioid-induced pruritus unresponsive to antihistamines. *J Pain Symptom Manage* **12**:255–60.

42. Bernstein JE, Grinzi RA. (1981). Butorphanol-induced pruritus antagonized by naloxone. *J Am Acad Dermatol* **5**:227–8.

43. Kamei J, Nagase H. (2001). Norbinaltorphimine, a selective kappa-opioid receptor antagonist, induces an itch-associated response in mice. *Eur J Pharmacol* **418**:141–5.

44. Stein H, Bijak M, Heerd E, *et al.* (1996). Pruritometer 1: portable measuring system for quantifying scratching as an objective measure of cholestatic pruritus. *Biomed Tech (Berl)* **41**:248–52.

45. Charuluxananan S, Somboonviboon W, Kyokong O, Nimcharoendee K. (2000). Ondansetron for treatment of intrathecal morphine-induced pruritus after cesarean delivery. *Reg Anesth Pain Med* **25**:535–9.

46. Cadranel JF, Di Martino V, Devergie B. (1997). Grapefruit juice for the pruritus of cholestatic liver disease. *Ann Intern Med* **126**:920–1.

47. Yazigi A, Chalhoub V, Madi-Jebara S, Haddad F, Hayek G. (2002). Prophylactic ondansetron is effective in the treatment of nausea and vomiting but not on pruritus after cesarean delivery with intrathecal sufentanil–morphine. *J Clin Anesth* **14**:183–6.

48. Asokumar B, Newman LM, McCarthy RJ, Ivankovich AD, Tuman KJ. (1998). Intrathecal bupivacaine reduces pruritus and prolongs duration of fentanyl analgesia during labor: a prospective, randomized controlled trial. *Anesth Analg* **87**:1309–15.

49. Borgeat A, Wilder-Smith OH, Saiah M, Rifat K. (1992). Subhypnotic doses of propofol relieve pruritus induced by epidural and intrathecal morphine. *Anesthesiology* **76**:510–12.

50. Nightingale C. (1995). A new treatment for epidural opioid induced pruritis in parturients. *Anaesthesia* **50**:185.

51. Imboden E, Zurcher T. (1995). Reply to "So the itch remains bearable" 10/95. Treatment of eczema—the Bernese version. *Krankenpfl Soins Infirm* **88**:64–6.

52. Beilin Y, Bernstein HH, Zucker-Pinchoff B, Zahn J, Zenzen WJ. (1998). Subhypnotic doses of propofol do not relieve pruritus induced by intrathecal morphine after cesarean section. *Anesth Analg* **86**:310–13.

53. Warwick JP, Kearns CF, Scott WE. (1997). The effect of subhypnotic doses of propofol on the incidence of pruritus after intrathecal morphine for caesarean section. *Anaesthesia* **52**:270–5.

54. Ball AJ. (1997). Identifying the caudal space—if it doesn't itch don't scratch. *Anaesthesia* **52**:506.

55. Horta ML, Ramos L, Goncalves Zda R, *et al.* (1996). Inhibition of epidural morphine-induced pruritus by intravenous droperidol. The effect of increasing the doses of morphine and of droperidol. *Reg Anesth* **21**:312–7.

56. Carvalho JC, Mathias RS, Senra WG, *et al.* (1991). Systemic droperidol and epidural morphine in the management of postoperative pain. *Anesth Analg* **72**:416.

57. Nakata K, Mammoto T, Kita T, et al. (2002). Continuous epidural, not intravenous, droperidol inhibits pruritus, nausea, and vomiting during epidural morphine analgesia. *J Clin Anesth* **14**:121–5.

58. Gage JC, D'Angelo R, Miller R, Eisenach JC. (1997). Does dextrose affect analgesia or the side effects of intrathecal sufentanil? *Anesth Analg* **85**:826–30.

59. Abouleish AE, Portnoy D, Abouleish EI. (2000). Addition of dextrose 3.5% to intrathecal sufentanil for labour analgesia reduces pruritus. *Can J Anaesth* **47**: 1171–5.

60. Gurkan Y, Toker K. (2002). Prophylactic ondansetron reduces the incidence of intrathecal fentanyl-induced pruritus. *Anesth Analg* **95**:1763–6, table of contents.

61. Henry A, Tetzlaff JE, Steckner K. (2002). Ondansetron is effective in treatment of pruritus after intrathecal fentanyl. *Reg Anesth Pain Med* **27**:538–40.

62. Thomas DA, Williams GM, Iwata K, Kenshalo DR Jr, Dubner R. (1993). Multiple effects of morphine on facial scratching in monkeys. *Anesth Analg* **77**:933–5.

63. McLelland J. (1986). The mechanism of morphine-induced urticaria. *Arch Dermatol* **122**:138–9.

64. Rosow CE, Moss J, Philbin DM, Savarese JJ. (1982). Histamine release during morphine and fentanyl anesthesia. *Anesthesiology* **56**:93–6.

65. Klinker JF, Seifert R. (1997). Morphine and muscle relaxants are receptor-independent G-protein activators and cromolyn is an inhibitor of stimulated G-protein activity. *Inflamm Res* **46**:46–50.

66. Wright DG, Thompson EM, Mathews H. (1993). Pruritus, PCAs and pain after caesarean section. *Anaesthesia* **48**:449–50.

67. Katcher J, Walsh D. (1999). Opioid-induced itching: morphine sulfate and hydromorphone hydrochloride. *J Pain Symptom Manage* **17**:70–2.

68. Woodham M. (1988). Pruritus with sublingual buprenorphine. *Anaesthesia* **43**: 806–7.

69. Krause L, Shuster S. (1983). Mechanism of action of antipruritic drugs. *Br Med J (Clin Res Ed)* **287**:1199–200.

70. Zylicz Z, Smits C, Krajnik M. (1998). Paroxetine for pruritus in advanced cancer. *J Pain Symptom Manage* **16**:121–4.

71. Crighton IM, Hobbs GJ, Reid MF. (1996). Ondansetron for the treatment of pruritus after spinal opioids. *Anaesthesia* **51**:199–200.

72. Kyriakides K, Hussain SK, Hobbs GJ. (1999). Management of opioid-induced pruritus: a role for 5-HT$_3$ antagonists? *Br J Anaesth* **82**:439–41.

8

Pruritus accompanying solid tumours

Małgorzata Krajnik and Zbigniew Zylicz

Pruritus in cancer: the phenomenon

Apart from lymphoproliferative and haematological disorders, that are frequently associated with pruritus (see Chapter 9), pruritus in patients with cancer is uncommon. It may complicate malignant diseases in four different ways:

- pruritus as a consequence of tumour growth;
- pruritus secondary to cholestasis;
- central pruritus caused by brain tumours;
- pruritus as complication of treatment.

Pruritus as a consequence of tumour growth

Paraneoplastic pruritus

Generalized pruritus may be the presenting symptom of a solid tumour, and may be present for several years before the diagnosis is made.[1–5] As a paraneoplastic symptom, it has been reported in patients with malignant tumours of the breast, stomach, lung, prostate, uterus, colon, nasopharynx, larynx, and others.[1, 6] Occasionally, the malignant disease is associated with a specific, recognizable dermatosis, for example, pemphigus[7–10] or bullous pemphigoid.[11–14] However, a study of 497 patients with bullous pemphigoid and positive immunofluorescence test did not reveal an increased incidence of cancer.[15]

The pathophysiology of paraneoplastic pruritus in malignant disease is not known. One of the oldest hypotheses suggests an allergic reaction of the host to the tumour-specific antigens.[16] In 1942 Urbach believed that products of cancer tissue could activate histamine with resultant widespread urticaria.[17] However, a subsequent study indicated that cancer patients have a low sensitivity to histamine-induced pruritus and antihistamines are not effective in relieving paraneoplastic pruritus.[18] It has also been suggested that pruritus may result from toxic products of necrotic tumour cells entering the systemic circulation and that pruritus might be due to an immune response indicated by microscopic cutaneous deposits of tumour. In some patients, pruritus may be due to non-specific debilitating effects of cancer that make the skin more susceptible to external irritants.

Pruritus may be prominent in paraneoplastic neuropathy, which occasionally complicates breast cancer.[19] The syndrome is characterized by upper and lower extremity paraesthesias and numbness, itching, muscle weakness, and cramps. In some patients radicular symptoms and signs are present. In some cases neuropathy was present up to 8 years before the diagnosis of breast cancer.[19] There are several reports of notalgia paraesthetica, localized pruritus of the upper midback, associated with multiple endocrine neoplasia type 2A.[20] Brachioradial pruritus caused by spinal cord tumour (ependymoma) has also been described.[21]

Pruritus secondary to cholestasis

Most often the pruritus is secondary to cholestasis caused by carcinoma of the pancreas head. The pathophysiology of this type of pruritus may be comparable if not identical to that of pruritus occurring in non-malignant chronic liver diseases (see Chapter 5). However, after placing a stent in the common bile duct, pruritus does not always disappear, suggesting that pruritus, at least in some cases of jaundiced patients with pancreatic cancer, is a paraneoplastic phenomenon.

Central pruritus caused by brain tumours

In some advanced brain tumours pruritus occurs and is characteristically restricted to the nostrils. Paroxysmal facial itch may be associated with brainstem glioma.[16] Pruritus of the nostrils is usually severe and persistent, and the patient scratches even during sleep. Unilateral cerebral lesions such as cerebral tumours and cerebrovascular lesions can be associated with pruritus probably through relief of central inhibition of pruritus.[22, 23] Pruritus caused by a brain tumour is usually contralateral to the lesion and may be accompanied by other sensory abnormalities. Tumours invading the fourth ventricle are specifically associated with (facial) pruritus.

Pruritus as a complication of treatment

Patients treated with surgery or receiving radiotherapy, cytotoxic chemotherapy, and/or biological response modifiers for treatment of malignancy are likely to experience pruritus.[24] Also, nerve damage induced by surgery may lead to pruritus in sensitive patients.

Surgery

Breast amputation is most often complicated by post-mastectomy pain. Occasionally, this neuropathy may be experienced as severe pruritus. Although there are no reports in the literature, three cases of severe pruritus after mastectomy have been observed by the authors. In two of these three cases, there was a history of long-standing pruritus associated with atopic dermatitis in childhood. It is possible, that the neural system is pre-conditioned by atopic dermatitis and more C-fibres are recruited for transmission of pruritic impulses. Damage of the nerves in such patients may result in neuropathic pruritus, but not pain (see Chapter 10).

Radiotherapy

Radiotherapy can provoke local acute or chronic radiodermatitis. Of women receiving radiotherapy for different tumours, 17% developed pruritic eruptions predominantly on the lower extremities.[25] Careful skin care is necessary to avoid ulceration, pain, and pruritus.[26, 27] Because of its unique presentation, the term 'eosinophilic, polymorphic, and pruritic eruption associated with radiotherapy' (EPPER) was proposed.[25] The heterogeneity of its clinical and histopathological manifestations suggests that EPPER may represent a spectrum of lesions involving cutaneous immune reactions. Radiotherapy may precipitate a cascade of events mediated by different cytokines, specific T lymphocytes, or both that leads to tissue damage by eosinophil-derived proteins. This syndrome may occur many months after starting radiotherapy.[28]

Chemotherapy

Each of the major classes of antineoplastic agents may elicit cutaneous reactions, including pruritus. Patients treated with chemotherapy often report itchy, dry skin and scaling that may be related to effects on sebaceous and sweat glands.[29] Most patients recover from this condition within weeks. Neuropathy (see Chapter 10), which may be generalized or segmental, may be more persistent. Some patients developed severe pruritus attributable to paclitaxel.[30] In this report pruritus had the features of neuropathy: it started after 1–3 cycles, with onset 1–14 days following the first infusion, and it lasted for 3–14 days. It started in the hands and feet and subsequently became more diffuse. In some patients itch was generalized from the beginning. Itch was accompanied by sensory neuropathy and symptoms such as tingling, burning, numbness, and pain were perceived at the same sites as the pruritus. Examination revealed decreased temperature sensation, allodynia, reduction of reflexes, and muscle weakness. In most patients pruritus decreased with administration of amitryptyline. Paclitaxel-induced generalized pruritus is a dose-dependent toxic effect. It is observed in only 13% of patients who were started on paclitaxel 175 mg/m². Its incidence increases to 58% of patients when the starting dose was 225 mg/m².[31]

Generalized pruritus may be a symptom of hypersensitivity reactions to chemotherapy.[32] It occurred in 17% of patients treated with carboplatin IV, but only a few of these discontinued treatment because of pruritus.[33] Most frequently, the intensity of pruritus decreases after administration of H_1-antihistamines (e.g. diphenhydramine) or corticosteroids. Pruritus has also been reported after intravesical cisplatin and mitomycin C.[34, 35] Perianal pruritus may be an underreported adverse effect of chemotherapy, especially gemcitabine.[36]

Miscellaneous

Among unexplained symptoms, perianal[37–39] and vulvovaginal[40] pruritus have been reported after intravenous bolus administration of a high dose of dexamethasone. Among other drugs used in oncology that may cause pruritus are megestrol acetate,[41] amifostine,[42] and recombinant cytokine therapy.[43] Spinal opioids used for the treatment of pain may also induce pruritus (see Chapter 7).

Evaluation and diagnosis

Pruritus caused by malignancy may precede the diagnosis by weeks or months, or occasionally years. It disappears rapidly when the cancer is successfully treated. Its reappearance may herald tumour recurrence.[44] Pruritus due to cancer usually differs from that encountered in lymphoma (see Chapter 9). Itching associated with cancer may be generalized or localized, it may occur preferentially in the pretibial areas, inner aspects of the thighs, upper thorax, shoulders, and the extensor surfaces of the upper extremities. Its intensity may change over time and there are no associated primary skin lesions. Sporadically, pruritus associated with solid tumours may present as aquagenic pruritus.[45]

Studies of patients with chronic generalized pruritus have not documented an increased incidence of cancers, but have revealed more cases of lymphoproliferative diseases, especially Hodgkin's disease, than expected.[44] Thus, in the absence of other systemic complaints or physical findings and after other benign and systemic causes have been excluded, the work-up should be directed first toward detecting a lymphoproliferative disease. Because pruritus may precede malignancy, if the initial evaluation of a patient with generalized pruritus does not reveal a malignancy, it is advisable to re-evaluate the patient periodically, for example, every 6 months.[3, 46]

Recognizing patterns

If pruritus is localized, it is unlikely to be related to malignancy. However, there are some exceptions. Vulval pruritus has been reported in patients with cancer of the cervix. Persistent pruritus in the scrotal and perineal region may be the first manifestation of prostate cancer. Perianal pruritus may accompany rectal or sigmoid cancer, and patients with this symptom should be vigilantly assessed to exclude the diagnosis of colorectal cancer.[47] The diagnosis of Paget's perianal disease should be considered in any patient with perianal pruritus and a rash, that does not respond to conventional therapy within a month.[48] In 33–86% of reported cases of Paget's perianal disease there is an associated underlying visceral cancer.[48–51] Patients with this condition should be thoroughly investigated for associated gastrointestinal malignancies. Cutaneous metastases, particularly in *en cuirass* breast cancer, are sometimes both painful and itchy. This type of itch may respond to nonsteroidal anti-inflammatory drugs (NSAIDs).[52]

Localized pruritus due to malignancy may resemble neuropathy (see Chapter 10). Patients with neurofibromatosis sometimes have localized or generalized pruritus. An infant with features of neurofibromatosis, presenting with symptoms of a spinal cord tumour including symmetrical pruritus of a characteristic dermatomal distribution, was described.[53] Pruritus in neurofibromatosis may be problematic. Some authors have suggested a role of localized chronic secretions from mast cells. In a controlled trial ketotifen, a mast cell stabilizer, and H_1-antihistamines decreased both pruritus and pain in patients with neurofibromatosis.[54] In several patients, neurofibromatosis and pruritus were associated with a brainstem glioma.[55]

Treatment

Treatment of pruritus caused by cancer should primarily be directed at the underlying malignant disease. However, in terminally ill patients, a symptomatic approach should prevail. For pruritus and jaundice due to carcinoma of the head of the pancreas, the stenting of the common bile duct is the treatment of choice. In many centres there is a huge experience with this procedure. The procedure is well tolerated. With the advent of premedication with midazolam, patients do not remember the procedure. Pain and bacteraemia may occur when the stent is occluded. Patients should come back to the hospital as soon as symptoms of biliary obstruction recur. The aim is to replace an occluded stent as soon as possible. Antibiotics may be given, but are probably not important. Infection clears up as soon as biliary obstruction is relieved. However, in palliative care we frequently see patients with occluded common bile duct stents. They frequently choose not to undergo a new procedure. In these patients, if the symptoms of septicaemia are not predominant, cholestasis and liver failure may progress rapidly. The patient may die before recurrence of pruritus. If pruritus is troublesome and the patient cannot take medication orally, the authors frequently use tropisetron, 1 or 2 mg subcutaneously p.r.n. This medication is highly effective, but also sedative.

Pharmacological interventions

Paraneoplastic itch associated with solid tumours is usually not eased by corticosteroids or cimetidine. However, paroxetine is almost always beneficial, often within 24–48 hours of starting therapy.[56] If paroxetine is not effective, it may be worthwhile to try mirtazapine 7.5–30 mg o.n.[57] It has been suggested that thalidomide may be efficacious in refractory paraneoplastic itch. The controlled trial of thalidomide involved patients with uraemic itch, but it may be relevant to paraneoplastic itch.[58] The effect of thalidomide seemed to be related to its capacity to reduce TNFα synthesis by monocytes and its anti-inflammatory properties.

Conclusions

- Paraneoplastic pruritus is a rare phenomenon, that is not yet widely recognized.
- Treatment of pruritus complicating cancer should be directed at the underlying maligancy.
- The most common pathogenesis of pruritus in cancer is cholestasis due to cancer of the head of the pancreas.
- The opioidergic tone in the brain is implicated in pruritus complicating cholestasis.
- Localized pruritus can be a sign of brain or spinal cord tumour.
- Radiotherapy and chemotherapy may cause transient or persistent pruritus.
- Paroxetine is the drug of choice for symptomatic treatment of pruritus complicating cancer.

References

1. Cormia FE. (1965). Pruritus, an uncommon but important symptom of systemic carcinoma. *Arch Dermatol* **92**:36–9.
2. Storck H. (1976). Cutaneous paraneoplastic syndromes. *Med Klin* **71**:356–72.
3. Lober CW. (1993). Pruritus and malignancy. *Clin Dermatol* **11**:125–8.
4. Beeaff DE. (1980). Pruritus as a sign of systemic disease. Report of metastatic small cell carcinoma. *Ariz Med* **37**:831–3.
5. Thomas S, Harrington CI. (1983). Intractable pruritus as the presenting symptom of carcinoma of the bronchus: a case report and review of the literature. *Clin Exp Dermatol* **8**:459–61.
6. Zirwas MJ, Seraly MP. (2001). Pruritus of unknown origin: a retrospective study. *J Am Acad Dermatol* **45**:892–6.
7. Ota M, Sato-Matsumura KC, Matsumura T, Tsuji Y, Ohkawara A. (2000). Pemphigus foliaceus and figurate erythema in a patient with prostate cancer. *Br J Dermatol* **142**:816–18.
8. Sherer Y, Shoenfeld Y. (1999). A malignancy work-up in patients with cancer-associated (paraneoplastic) autoimmune diseases: pemphigus and myasthenic syndromes as cases in point. *Oncol Rep* **6**:665–8.
9. Kubota Y, Yoshino Y, Mizoguchi M. (1994). A case of herpetiform pemphigus associated with lung cancer. *J Dermatol* **21**:609–11.
10. Choinzonov EL, Kitsmaniuk ZD, Oksenov BS. (1991). Laryngeal cancer developing in a patient with pemphigus vulgaris. *Vestn Otorinolaringol* **6**:59–60.

11. Egan CA, Lazarova Z, Darling TN, Yee C, Cote T, Yancey KB. (2001). Anti-epiligrin cicatricial pemphigoid and relative risk for cancer. *Lancet* **357**:1850–1.

12. Yamamoto T, Tanaka A, Furuse Y. (1994). Bullous pemphigoid with esophageal cancer. *J Dermatol* **21**:283–4.

13. Ikai K, Imamura S, Ogino A, Danno K, Hayakawa M. (1978). Bullous pemphigoid and metastatic skin cancer. *Dermatologica* **156**:55–8.

14. Thomas DA, Williams GM, Iwata K, Kenshalo DR Jr, Dubner R. (1992). Effects of central administration of opioids on facial scratching in monkeys. *Brain Res* **585**:315–17.

15. Lindelof B, Islam N, Eklund G, Arfors L. (1990). Pemphigoid and cancer. *Arch Dermatol* **126**:66–8.

16. Andreev VC, Petkov I. (1975). Skin manifestations associated with tumours of the brain. *Br J Dermatol* **92**:675–8.

17. Urbach E. (1942). Endogenous allergy. *Arch Derm Syph* **45**:697.

18. Burtin C, Noirot C, Giroux C, Scheinmann P. (1986). Decreased skin response to intradermal histamine in cancer patients . *J Allergy Clin Immunol* **78**:83–9.

19. Peterson K, Forsyth PA, Posner JB. (1994). Paraneoplastic sensorimotor neuropathy associated with breast cancer. *J Neurooncol* **21**:159–70.

20. Bugalho MJ, Limbert E, Sobrinho LG, *et al.* (1992). A kindred with multiple endocrine neoplasia type 2A associated with pruritic skin lesions. *Cancer* **70**:2664–7.

21. Kavak A, Dosoglu M. (2002). Can a spinal cord tumor cause brachioradial pruritus? *J Am Acad Dermatol* **46**:437–40.

22. Massey EW. (1984). Unilateral neurogenic pruritus following stroke. *Stroke* **15**:901–3.

23. Sullivan MJ, Drake ME Jr. (1984). Unilateral pruritus and *Nocardia* brain abscess. *Neurology* **34**:828–9.

24. Cortina P, Garrido JA, Tomas JF, Unamuno P, Armijo M. (1990). 'Flagellate' erythema from bleomycin. With histopathological findings suggestive of inflammatory oncotaxis. *Dermatologica* **180**:106–9.

25. Rueda RA, Valencia IC, Covelli C, *et al.* (1999). Eosinophilic, polymorphic, and pruritic eruption associated with radiotherapy. *Arch Dermatol* **135**:804–10.

26. Lokkevik E, Skovlund E, Reitan JB, Hannisdal E, Tanum G. (1996). Skin treatment with bepanthen cream versus no cream during radiotherapy—a randomized controlled trial. *Acta Oncol* **35**:1021–6.

27. Lavery BA. (1995). Skin care during radiotherapy: a survey of UK practice. *Clin Oncol (R Coll Radiol)* **7**:184–7.

28. Gallego H, Crutchfield CE 3rd, Wilke MS, Lewis EJ. (2001). Delayed EPPER syndrome. *Arch Dermatol* **137**:821–2.

29. Hood AF. (1986). Cutaneous side effects of cancer chemotherapy. *Med Clin North Am* **70**:187–209.

30. Freilich RJ, Seidman AD. (1995). Pruritis caused by 3-hour infusion of high-dose paclitaxel and improvement with tricyclic antidepressants. *J Natl Cancer Inst* **87**:933–4.

31. Gianni L, Munzone E, Capri G, *et al.* (1995). Paclitaxel in metastatic breast cancer: a trial of two doses by a 3-hour infusion in patients with disease recurrence after prior therapy with anthracyclines. *J Natl Cancer Inst* **87**:1169–75.

32. Alkins SA, Byrd JC, Morgan SK, Ward FT, Weiss RB. (1996). Anaphylactoid reactions to methotrexate. *Cancer* **77**:2123–6.

33. Polyzos A, Tsavaris N, Kosmas C, *et al.* (2001). Hypersensitivity reactions to carboplatin administration are common but not always severe: a 10-year experience. *Oncology* **61**:129–33.

34. Blumenreich MS, Needles B, Yagoda A, Sogani P, Grabstald H, Whitmore WF Jr. (1982). Intravesical cisplatin for superficial bladder tumors. *Cancer* **50**:863–5.

35. Kunkeler L, Nieboer C, Bruynzeel DP. (2000). Type III and type IV hypersensitivity reactions due to mitomycin C. *Contact Dermatitis* **42**:74–6.

36. Hejna M, Valencak J, Raderer M. (1999). Anal pruritus after cancer chemotherapy with gemcitabine. *N Engl J Med* **340**:655–6.

37. Klygis LM. (1992). Dexamethasone-induced perineal irritation in head injury. *Am J Emerg Med* **10**:268.

38. Andrews D, Grunau VJ. (1986). An uncommon adverse effect following bolus administration of intravenous dexamethasone. *J Can Dent Assoc* **52**:309–11.

39. Czerwinski AW, Czerwinski AB, Whitsett TL, Clark ML. (1972). Effects of a single, large, intravenous injection of dexamethasone. *Clin Pharmacol Ther* **13**:638–42.

40. Taleb N, Geahchan N, Ghosn M, Brihi E, Sacre P. (1988). Vulvar pruritus after high-dose dexamethasone. *Eur J Cancer Clin Oncol* **24**:495.

41. Brufman G, Isacson R, Haim N, Gez E, Sulkes A. (1994). Megestrol acetate in advanced breast carcinoma after failure to tamoxifen and/or amino-glutethimide. *Oncology* **51**:258–61.

42. Shaw PJ, Bleakley M. (2000). Systemic inflammatory response syndrome associated with amifostine. *Med Pediatr Oncol* **34**:309–10.

43. Asnis LA, Gaspari AA. (1995). Cutaneous reactions to recombinant cytokine therapy. *J Am Acad Dermatol* **33**:393–410.

44. Goldman BD, Koch HK. (1994). Pruritus and malignancy. In: Bernhard JD. (ed.), *Itch. Mechanisms and management of pruritus*, New York: McGraw-Hill, pp. 299–319.

45. Ferguson JE, August PJ, Guy AJ. (1994). Aquagenic pruritus associated with metastatic squamous cell carcinoma of the cervix. *Clin Exp Dermatol* **19**:257–8.

46. Lober CW. (1988). Should the patient with generalized pruritus be evaluated for malignancy? *J Am Acad Dermatol* **19**:350–2.

47. Pfenninger JL, Zainea GG. (2001). Common anorectal conditions: Part I. Symptoms and complaints. *Am Fam Physician* **63**:2391–8.

48. Khoubehi B, Schofield A, Leslie M, Slevin ML, Talbot IC, Northover JM. (2001). Metastatic in-situ perianal Paget's disease. *J R Soc Med* **94**:137–8.

49. Redondo P, Idoate M, Espana A, Quintanilla E. (1995). Pruritus ani in an elderly man. Extramammary Paget's disease. *Arch Dermatol* **131**:952–3, 955–6.

50. Eusebio EB, Graham J, Mody N. (1990). Treatment of intractable pruritus ani. *Dis Colon Rectum* **33**:770–2.

51. Powell FC, Perry HO. (1985). Pruritus ani: could it be malignant? *Geriatrics* **40**:89–91.

52. Twycross RG. (1981). Pruritus and pain in en cuirass breast cancer. *Lancet* **2**:696.

53. Johnson RE, Kanigsberg ND, Jimenez CL. (2000). Localized pruritus: a presenting symptom of a spinal cord tumor in a child with features of neurofibromatosis. *J Am Acad Dermatol* **43**:958–61.

54. Riccardi VM. (1993). A controlled multiphase trial of ketotifen to minimize neurofibroma-associated pain and itching. *Arch Dermatol* **129**:577–81.

55. Summers CG, MacDonald JT. (1988). Paroxysmal facial itch: a presenting sign of childhood brainstem glioma. *J Child Neurol* **3**:189–92.

56. Zylicz Z, Smits C, Krajnik M. (1998). Paroxetine for pruritus in advanced cancer. *J Pain Symptom Manage* **16**:121–4.

57. Davis MP, Frandsen JL, Walsh D, Andresen S, Taylor S. (2003). Mirtazapine for pruritus. *J Pain Symptom Manage* **25**:288–91.

58. Silva SR, Viana PC, Lugon NV, Hoette M, Ruzany F, Lugon JR. (1994). Thalidomide for the treatment of uremic pruritus: a crossover randomized double-blind trial. *Nephron* **67**:270–3.

9

Pruritus in haematological disorders

Małgorzata Krajnik and Zbigniew Zylicz

The magnitude of the problem

In contrast to solid tumours, pruritus is a frequent symptom in patients with haematological disorders. It is a significant problem in polycythaemia vera, Hodgkin's lymphoma, Sezary's syndrome (T-cell lymphoma), and occasionally also in leukaemia, multiple myeloma, Waldenström's macroglobinaemia, mycosis fungoides, benign gammopathy, and systemic mastocytosis. Pruritus may be the presenting symptom, but most often it is associated with advanced disease.[1–4]

Generalized pruritus occurs in nearly 50% of patients with polycythaemia vera. It occurs in about 30% of patients with Hodgkin's lymphoma, and may persist after remission of the disease.[5, 6] Itch is rare in non-Hodgkin's lymphoma, but its incidence is almost 100% in the rare Sezary's syndrome (T-cell lymphoma). The association between iron deficiency and pruritus is unexplained.[7] Pruritus affects only a minority of iron-deficient patients and does not correlate with the severity of the anaemia.

Polycythaemia vera and aquagenic pruritus

About 30–50% of patients with polycythaemia vera have a specific type of pruritus, called aquagenic pruritus. Although most patients with aquagenic pruritus are otherwise healthy, this type of pruritus may precede development of polycythaemia vera by several years.[8] Aquagenic pruritus is characterized by intense itching, sometimes accompanied by a burning or stinging sensation after contact with water. In aquagenic pruritus there are no cutaneous sensory alterations.[9, 10] Apart from polycythaemia vera, it may accompany other proliferative disorders, or be an isolated symptom. The discomfort occurs 1–5 minutes after exposure to water and lasts for 10–120 minutes. The triggering factor seems to be a sudden decrease in skin temperature. Humoral factors may be released or activated in the skin when it is cooled down.[11] After contact of the skin with water, increased degranulation of mast cells has been demonstrated and there may be release of acetylcholine[9] and/or histamine.[12]

Treatment

The use of interferon-α as a cytoreductive agent in polycythaemia vera is associated with amelioration of pruritus[13, 14] and should always be considered first.[15] Pruritus in polycythaemia vera appears to be associated with raised histamine concentrations in blood and urine, but H_1-antihistamines, are usually ineffective. Cyproheptadine was the only antihistamine to be effective in decreasing pruritus, but it is also a strong antagonist of serotonin.[16] Pizotifen, a potent antihistaminic and antiserotoninergic drug, prescribed for migraine prophylaxis, also had antipruritic effect in polycythaemia vera.[17] There have been some reports of benefit with cimetidine, but its role is not yet established.[8] Pruritus in polycythaemia vera often responds well to paroxetine.[18, 19] However, the drug of choice is low-dose aspirin: 300 mg is usually effective within 30 min, and its effect lasts for 12–24 hours.[20] Platelet degranulation is increased in polycythaemia vera with release of serotonin and prostanoids. This degranulation is known to be decreased by aspirin and the antipruritic effect of aspirin could be related to its impact on platelet dynamics. However, Fjellner and Hägermark[11] found no functional abnormality of platelets and proposed a mechanism for enhanced platelet aggregation in polycythaemia vera. They proposed that, when the skin is cooled down, adenosine diphosphate (ADP) from erythrocytes and catecholamines released from adrenergic vasoconstrictor nerves might stimulate platelets to aggregate in skin vessels and to produce and release pruritogens, prostaglandin E_2 (PgE_2), and serotonin.[11]

Topical scopolamine inhibits pruritus after contact with water, but it is not efficacious for generalized pruritus. Increased cutaneous fibrinolytic activity has been demonstrated both before and after contact of skin with water.[21] The effectiveness of topical capsaicin treatment suggests that substance P and other neuropeptides released from cutaneous nerve fibres play a key role in mediating aquagenic pruritus.[22] Psoralen plus ultraviolet A

(PUVA) treatment may also be helpful in aquagenic pruritus, probably by leading to a reduction of responsiveness of cutaneous sensory nerves, similar to that observed after topical capsaicin.[23] Addition of baking soda to bath water to raise the pH to 8 may be helpful, but at least 0.5 kg is needed for an average bath.[23] Colestyramine is effective in the treatment of pruritus in polycythaemia vera, probably by extracting substances other than bile salts.[24] Correction of venesection-induced iron deficiency may also give relief, but should be done carefully as it may cause an exacerbation of polycythaemia vera.[15]

Lymphoproliferative disorders

Hodgkin's disease

Pruritus occurs in about 30% of patients with Hodgkin's lymphoma.[25] It may precede the diagnosis of the disease by as much as 5 years.[26, 27] It is often worse at night and it starts in the legs and later extends all over the body.[28] Generalized pruritus tends to occur more often in the nodular sclerosis type of Hodgkin's disease associated with a mediastinal mass.[25] In localized disease pruritus tends to occur in the area drained by lymphatic vessels invaded by the disease. Generalized pruritus was considered to be a B symptom of Hodgkin's disease from 1965 till 1971 but, following several studies showing that pruritus had a negligible impact on survival, was replaced by the weight loss.[25] However, later reports suggested that patients with Hodgkin's lymphoma, mycosis fungoides, and severe pruritus did less well than stage-matched non-pruritic patients.[29] Based on these and other studies, severe pruritus was found to be more important than night sweats in identifying patients who require more aggressive therapy.

Histamine has been suggested as an important pruritogen in generalized pruritus associated with lymphoproliferative diseases. It may be released from basophils, which are usually increased in number. The activity of histidine decarboxylase, which is responsible for the production of histamine, is elevated in these cells.[30] In Hodgkin's disease it has been suggested that an autoimmune response to lymphoid cells may cause release of pruritogens such as leukopeptidases and bradykinin.[25] The eosinophilia seen in the pleomorphic infiltrate of Hodgkin's disease may be linked to histamine release, and a role for high serum levels of IgE has been proposed.[31] Specific cutaneous deposits occur in 10–20% of patients with lymphoma or leukaemia. With the exception of uncommon cutaneous nodular lesions in Hodgkin's disease, which are usually pruritic, the lesions in leukaemia and other lymphomas are usually asymptomatic, but may induce a burning sensation, rather than pruritus. The presence of specific skin lesions is believed to be a poor prognostic sign.[31] About 5–10% of patients with Hodgkin's lymphoma become clinically jaundiced. Occasionally, jaundice is caused by hepatic involvement with lymphoma. Alternatively it may be caused by intrahepatic cholestasis due to vanishing bile duct syndrome.[32] How much of the pruritus of Hodgkin's lymphoma is due to hepatic infiltration and cholestasis is unclear. At autopsy, the incidence of hepatic involvement with lymphoma is over 50%.

Treatment

Treatment of pruritus complicating Hodgkin's disease is best accomplished by treating the lymphoma. If this fails there is no standard therapy. Cimetidine has been shown to be an effective symptomatic treatment.[33] The pruritogens in Hodgkin's disease may be different to those in other pruritic conditions. Stimulation of H_2 receptors may cause pruritus in Hodgkin's disease but not in other conditions. Corticosteroids often relieve pruritus in late-stage Hodgkin's lymphoma; the mechanism of this effect is unknown. However, this traditional treatment is not supported by any published evidence. In the past some patients appeared to derive benefit from γ-interferon, but this treatment is no longer used.[29] In general there are three treatment steps:

- treatment of the Hodgkin's lymphoma;
- trial of corticosteroids;
- cimetidine 800 mg/24 hours.

If there is pruritus, cholestasis, and the vanishing bile duct syndrome, an opioid antagonist such as naltrexone should be tried.

Of course, if the patient needs gastric mucosal protection while receiving corticosteroids, cimetidine should be the drug of choice. In refractory cases mirtazapine 7.5–30 mg o.n. may be tried.[34]

Cutaneous T cell lymphomas

Cutaneous T cell lymphomas occur in middle-aged adults, particularly males. Major variants include mycosis fungoides and Sezary syndrome. One of the constant characteristics of both of these variants is severe pruritus. The early phase of mycosis fungoides is characterized by the presence of a chronic non-specific dermatitis that is frequently associated with pruritus[26, 35] and lymphadenopathy.[25] Although generalized pruritus does not usually occur in the absence of cutaneous manifestations, it may precede cutaneous manifestations of the disease by up to 10 years. Mycosis fungoides should be suspected in any patient with dermatitis and severe pruritus. There are some reports of 'invisible' mycosis fungoides, which is manifested by severe pruritus in the absence of any visible cutaneous lesions.[35, 36] In such cases it is advisable to undertake random skin biopsies of normally looking skin; such biopsies may establish a histological diagnosis of mycosis fungoides. In mycosis fungoides pruritus appears to be associated with the degree of histological epidermotropism of the neoplastic and inflammatory cells infiltrations. Release of pruritogens close to the dermo-epidermal nerve endings may lead to pruritus. Others have proposed that pruritus in mycosis fungoides may be due to release of leukopeptidases and cellular products due to host resistance to the malignant cells.[37] In Sezary syndrome, the pruritus may be due to the production and release of soluble T-cell lymphokines, such as interleukin 2 (IL-2).[37] In advanced stages of both types of cutaneous T cell lymphoma, patients develop hepatic, splenic, gastrointestinal tract, pulmonary, and renal involvement. Infiltration of the bone marrow, circulating leukaemic cells, and generalized erythrodermia may make pruritus more severe.

Treatment

Mycosis fungoides cells are extremely sensitive to radiation-induced necrosis. Radiation therapy, topical nitrogen mustard, chemotherapy, PUVA, photophoresis, and other measures that act against the underlying tumour have been associated with symptomatic relief of pruritus.[35, 38] Cyclosporin A has been reported to relieve this type of pruritus rapidly, but little is known about its long-term effects on the disease.[37] Preparations containing menthol usually have satisfactory local antipruritic effects in mycosis fungoides. Again, corticosteroids are widely used in this disease also and appear to ameliorate pruritus, although formal studies confirming their efficacy have not been published.

Other lymphoproliferative disorders

The incidence and significance of pruritus in other lymphomas and leukaemias is unknown. This symptom has been reported in approximately 3% of patients with non-Hodgkin's lymphoma.[26] Intractable pruritus in non-Hodgkin's lymphoma has been reported; it did not decrease after chemotherapy but was rapidly ameliorated by interferon-α therapy.[39]

Pruritus more commonly occurs in lymphocytic than in granulocytic leukaemia and is more frequent in chronic rather than acute leukaemia.

Pruritus has been reported as a rare initial symptom in multiple myeloma, Waldenström's macroglobulinaemia, and some benign gammopathies.[40] In one report a patient with sun- and water-induced pruritus, associated with porphyria cutanea tarda, developed chronic myeloid leukaemia 3 years later.[41]

Iron deficiency

Pruritus caused by uncomplicated iron deficiency has been described in several reports.[42–45] However, most patients with severe iron deficiency anaemia never develop pruritus. Iron deficiency by itself, with or without anaemia, has occasionally been reported as a cause of generalized pruritus.[46] In women, the origins of iron deficiency may be different, but in men anaemia is most often associated with alcohol-related liver cirrhosis or unrecognized cancer. Generalized pruritus associated with iron deficiency, particularly in the elderly male, is cause for concern. Simple screening procedures, such as serum ferritin, faecal occult blood, and urinalysis, should be done as soon as possible. The pathogenesis of pruritus may be a direct result of iron deficiency that leads to psychological and epithelial changes. These changes may predispose to pruritus. Iron is necessary for the activity of many enzymes. Altered activities of enzymes may lead to metabolic disturbances and pruritus. Pruritus due to iron deficiency responds to iron therapy, which should be continued until the iron stores are restored. However, in polycythaemia vera, loading with iron may exacerbate the disease and lead to an unacceptably high and dangerous haematocrit.[44]

Should patients with generalized pruritus be screened and monitored for malignancy?

A study of 125 patients with generaliszed pruritus, who were followed for up to 6 years, did not show a significant overall increase in malignancies, except for lymphomas.[47] However, the numbers were small and the findings have not been confirmed by others. Nevertheless, a search for an occult malignancy in a patient with generalized pruritus should probably be directed only to lymphoproliferative disorders.[26] It is advisable, to investigate such patients periodically, for example, every 6 months. However, periodic screening may evoke feelings of anxiety and carcinophobia in some patients.

Conclusions

- Severe pruritus is experienced by many patients with polycythaemia vera.

- Cytoreductive treatment, together with aspirin and/or cimetidine, is advocated as the first-line treatment of pruritus in polycythaemia vera.

- Aquagenic pruritus is frequently associated with polycythaemia vera, although patients suffering from this type of pruritus alone should not be concerned about developing haematological disorders.

- Paroxetine may have an important place in the symptomatic treatment of pruritus in polycythaemia vera.

- Pruritus is a common feature of Hodgkin disease. Part of it may be secondary to intrahepatic cholestasis.

- Pruritus is very common in cutaneous T cell lymphomas.

- Treatment of pruritus in lymphoproliferative disorders should be directed at the underlying disease if possible.

- If cytoreductive treatment fails, pruritus in lymphoproliferative disorders may be treated with corticosteroids and/or cimetidine.

- Screening for occult haematological malignancy in patients with generalized pruritus of unestablished aetiology is not advocated for all patients. In some, such screening may do more harm than good.

References

1. Rajka G. (1966). Investigation of patients suffering from generalized pruritus, with special references to systemic diseases. *Acta Derm Venereol* **46**:190–4.

2. Fine J. (1980). Mastocytosis. *Int J Dermatol* **19**:117–23.

3. Abdel-Naser MB, Gollnick H, Orfanos CE. (1993). Aquagenic pruritus as a presenting symptom of polycythemia vera. *Dermatology* **187**:130–3.

4. Abel EA, Wood GS, Hoppe RT. (1993). Mycosis fungoides: clinical and histologic features, staging, evaluation, and approach to treatment. *CA Cancer J Clin* **43**:93–115.

5. Winkelmann RK. (1988). Pruritus. *Semin Dermatol* **7**:233–5.

6. Botero F. (1978). Pruritus as a manifestation of systemic disorders. *Cutis* **21**:873–80.

7. Lewiecki EM, Rahman F. (1976). Pruritus. A manifestation of iron deficiency. *J Am Med Assoc* **236**:2319–20.

8. Easton P, Galbraith PR. (1978). Cimetidine treatment of pruritus in polycythemia vera. *N Engl J Med* **299**:1134.

9. Greaves MW, Black AK, Eady RA, Coutts A. (1981). Aquagenic pruritus. *Br Med J (Clin Res Ed)* **282**:2008–10.

10. Steinman HK, Greaves MW. (1985). Aquagenic pruritus. *J Am Acad Dermatol* **13**:91–6.

11. Fjellner B, Hägermark O. (1979). Pruritus in polycythemia vera: treatment with aspirin and possibility of platelet involvement. *Acta Derm Venereol* **59**:505–12.

12. Steinman HK, Kobza-Black A, Lotti TM, Brunetti L, Panconesi E, Greaves MW. (1987). Polycythaemia rubra vera and water-induced pruritus: blood histamine levels and cutaneous fibrinolytic activity before and after water challenge. *Br J Dermatol* **116**:329–33.

13. Finelli C, Gugliotta L, Gamberi B, Vianelli N, Visani G, Tura S. (1993). Relief of intractable pruritus in polycythemia vera with recombinant interferon alfa. *Am J Hematol* **43**:316–18.

14. Muller EW, de Wolf JT, Egger R, *et al.* (1995). Long-term treatment with interferon-alpha 2b for severe pruritus in patients with polycythaemia vera. *Br J Haematol* **89**:313–18.

15. Tefferi A. (2003). Polycythemia vera: a comprehensive review and clinical recommendations. *Mayo Clin Proc* **78**:174–94.

16. Gilbert HS, Warner RR, Wasserman LR. (1966). A study of histamine in myeloproliferative disease. *Blood* **28**:795–806.

17. Fitzsimons EJ, Dagg JH, McAllister EJ. (1981). Pruritus of polycythaemia vera: a place for pizotifen? *Br Med J (Clin Res Ed)* **283**:277.

18. Diehn F, Tefferi A. (2001). Pruritus in polycythaemia vera: prevalence, laboratory correlates and management. *Br J Haematol* **115**:619–21.

19. Tefferi A, Fonseca R. (2002). Selective serotonin reuptake inhibitors are effective in the treatment of polycythemia vera-associated pruritus. *Blood* **99**:2627.

20. Jackson N, Burt D, Crocker J, Boughton B. (1987). Skin mast cells in polycythaemia vera: relationship to the pathogenesis and treatment of pruritus. *Br J Dermatol* **116**:21–9.

21. Lotti T, Steinman HK, Greaves MW, Fabbri P, Brunetti L, Panconesi E. (1986). Increased cutaneous fibrinolytic activity in aquagenic pruritus. *Int J Dermatol* **25**:508–10.

22. Lotti T, Teofoli P, Tsampau D. (1994). Treatment of aquagenic pruritus with topical capsaicin cream. *J Am Acad Dermatol* **30**:232–5.

23. Menage HD, Norris PG, Hawk JL, Graves MW. (1993). The efficacy of psoralen photochemotherapy in the treatment of aquagenic pruritus. *Br J Dermatol* **129**:163–5.

24. Chanarin I, Szur L. (1975). Relief of intractable pruritis in polycythaemia rubra vera with cholestyramine. *Br J Haematol* **29**:669–70.

25. Goldman BD, Koch HK. (1994). Pruritus and malignancy. In: Bernhard JD. (ed.), *Itch. Mechanisms and management of pruritus*, New York: McGraw-Hill, pp. 299–319.

26. Lober CW. (1988). Should the patient with generalized pruritus be evaluated for malignancy? *J Am Acad Dermatol* **19**:350–2.

27. O'Donnell BF, Alton B, Carney D, O'Loughlin S. (1993). Generalized pruritus: when to investigate further. *J Am Acad Dermatol* **28**:117.

28. Cavalli F. (1998). Rare syndromes in Hodgkin's disease. *Ann Oncol* **9** (Suppl. 5): S109–13.

29. Gobbi PG, Attardo-Parrinello G, Lattanzio G, Rizzo SC, Ascari E. (1983). Severe pruritus should be a B-symptom in Hodgkin's disease. *Cancer* **51**:1934–6.

30. Gilchrest BA. (1982). Pruritus: pathogenesis, therapy, and significance in systemic disease states. *Arch Intern Med* **142**:101–5.

31. Czarnecki DB, Downes NP, O'Brien T. (1982). Pruritic specific cutaneous infiltrates in leukemia and lymphoma. *Arch Dermatol* **118**:119–21.

32. Hubscher SG, Lumley MA, Elias E. (1993). Vanishing bile duct syndrome: a possible mechanism for intrahepatic cholestasis in Hodgkin's lymphoma. *Hepatology* **17**:70–7.

33. Aymard JP, Lederlin P, Witz F, Colomb JN, Herbeuval R, Weber B. (1980). Cimetidine for pruritus in Hodgkin's disease. *Br Med J* **280**:151–2.

34. Davis MP, Frandsen JL, Walsh D, Andresen S, Taylor S. (2003). Mirtazapine for pruritus. *J Pain Symptom Manage* **25**:288–91.

35. Pujol RM, Gallardo F, Llistosella E, *et al.* (2000). Invisible mycosis fungoides: a diagnostic challenge. *J Am Acad Dermatol* **42**:324–8.

36. Dereure O, Guilhou JJ. (2001). Invisible mycosis fungoides: a new case. *J Am Acad Dermatol* **45**:318–19.

37. Totterman TH, Scheynius A, Killander A, Danersund A, Alm GV. (1985). Treatment of therapy-resistant Sezary syndrome with cyclosporin-A: suppression of pruritus, leukaemic T cell activation markers and tumour mass. *Scand J Haematol* **34**:196–203.

38. Yamamoto T, Katayama I, Nishioka K. (1997). Role of mast cell and stem cell factor in hyperpigmented mycosis fungoides. *Blood* **90**:1338–40.

39. Radossi P, Tison T, Vianello F, Dazzi F. (1996). Intractable pruritus in non-Hodgkin lymphoma/CLL: rapid response to IFN alpha. *Br J Haematol* **94**:579.

40. Erskine JG, Rowan RM, Alexander JO, Sekoni GA. (1977). Pruritus as a presentation of myelomatosis. *Br Med J* **1**:687–8.

41. Granel B, Serratrice J, Bouabdallah R, *et al.* (2001). Atypical porphyria cutanea tarda in a patient with chronic myelogenous leukemia. *Dermatology* **203**:82–3.

42. Reeves JR. (1977). Iron-deficiency pruritus. *J Am Med Assoc* **237**:1435.

43. Takkunen H. (1978). Iron-deficiency pruritus. *J Am Med Assoc* **239**:1394.

44. Salem HH, Van der Weyden MB, Young IF, Wiley JS. (1982). Pruritus and severe iron deficiency in polycythaemia vera. *Br Med J (Clin Res Ed)* **285**:91–2.

45. Valsecchi R, Cainelli T. (1983). Generalized pruritus: a manifestation of iron deficiency. *Arch Dermatol* **119**:630.

46. Vickers CF. (1977). Iron-deficiency pruritus. *J Am Med Assoc* **238**:129.

47. Paul R, Paul R, Jansen CT. (1987). Itch and malignancy prognosis in generalized pruritus: a 6-year follow-up of 125 patients. *J Am Acad Dermatol* **16**:1179–82.

10

Neuropathic pruritus

Zbigniew Zylicz

The origin and classification of neuropathic pruritus

The term 'neurogenic pruritus' is used for pruritus originating anywhere in the central nervous system (CNS), as a result of neurotransmitters acting on the intact nervous system.[1] Neuropathy, implying nerve damage, can be subdivided into two types, specifically, degenerative and entrapment (Fig. 10.1). Degenerative neuropathy is more often diffuse and peripheral. The injured axons first degenerate and later regenerate. The regeneration process may be incomplete or aberrant, and may be associated with persistent sensory disorders, including pruritus. Usually, more than one nerve is affected (polyneuropathy). With nerve entrapment, initially the nerve may simply be dysfunctional but later it may degenerate. Initially, full recovery is possible. With degenerative neuropathy, hypo- or hypersensitivity in the itching area is prominent, whereas in entrapment neuropathy there are no disturbances of sensation and the pruritus is paroxysmal. Table 10.1 gives the definitions of some terms associated with neuropathic pruritus.

Symptomatology

In degenerative neuropathy pruritus is occasionally the sole symptom. It is usually localized rather than generalized, although the borders of the affected area may be ill-defined. In entrapment neuropathy the pruritus is limited to the area served by the affected cutaneous nerve (mononeuropathy). Entrapment usually involves proximal nerves, that is, those close to the spine, for example, root compression.

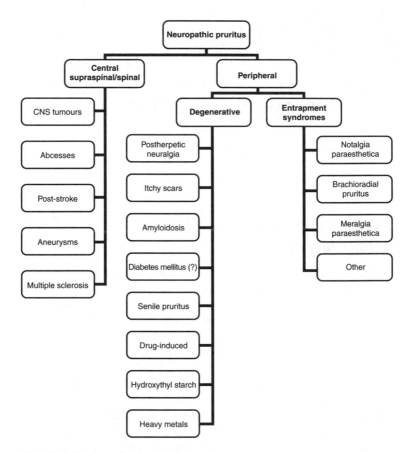

Fig. 10.1 Neuropathic pruritus.

In both types of neuropathy the predominant symptoms may be paraesthesia and pain. This symptom complex is called pruralgia. Patients may complain of 'pins-and-needles', tingling, stinging, or burning sensations. Pruritus may also be present, but is clearly only a part of the syndrome. The symptoms may elicit a desire to press on or rub the affected area, or to avoid light touch; only rarely do patients scratch. In the degenerative type there is a greater likelihood of allodynia and alloknesis. Other symptoms in the area of neuropathy may include aberrant temperature sensations, formication, and disturbance of sweating. Box 10.1 summarizes the characteristics of neuropathic pruritus.

Table 10.1 Terms and definitions

Neuropathy	A disturbance of function or pathological change in a nerve
Neuropathic pruritus	Pruritus caused by mechanisms interfering with pruritus transmission due to neuropathic changes
Neurogenic pruritus	Pruritus caused by mechanisms interfering with pruritus transmission in the healthy nervous system
Pruritic mediators	Pruritic mediators activate pruriceptors. In the CNS the mediators are no longer specific substances involved in transmission of pruritus in the second- and third-order neurons (e.g. glutamate is a neurotransmitter for pruritus, pain, touch, and warmth)
Pruralgia	Pruritus experienced together with pain
Allodynia	Pain caused by a stimulus that does not normally provoke pain
Alloknesis	Analogous to allodynia; touch-evoked pruritus
Hyperknesis	Strong response to a known pruritogenic factor
Polyneuropathy	Neuropathy affecting multiple peripheral nerves, e.g. when the cause is systemic
Mononeuropathy	Neuropathy affecting one single nerve, e.g. nerve entrapment
Formication	A form of paraesthesia or tactile hallucination. A sensation as if small insects were creeping under the skin (Latin: *formica* = ant)

It is important to differentiate between psychogenic pruritus (all of the above symptoms may be present!) and a neurological disorder (see Chapter 11).

The pathogenesis of the different types of peripheral neuropathy

Specific pruritus C-fibres are connected in large networks and have large innervation territories, up to 8.5 cm in diameter.[2] Damage to these very thin and vulnerable fibres may produce diffuse, localized pruritus. Damage may be local, for example, surgical injury or herpes zoster infection, or may be caused by systemic disease, for example, amyloidosis or uraemia. Although initially the damage is peripheral, it can lead to spontaneous

Box 10.1 Characteristics of neuropathic pruritus (according to John Y. Koo and Roger S. Lo)

- Delayed onset, for example, weeks or months
- Course of disease is usually chronic, but can be reversed with treatment of the CNS lesion
- Pruritus often localized to one side of the body, contralateral to the CNS lesion, or bilateral, in which case the onset is usually unilateral
- Pruritus may be accompanied by other sensory deficits
- Pruritus may be accompanied by anomalous sensory phenomenon such as dysaesthesia, allodynia, alloknesis, and hyperpathia
- Pruritic episodes may be precipitated by touch (alloknesis) or high temperature
- Pruritus is generally referred to cutaneous areas but may sometimes be restricted to the nostril and/or throat
- Pruritus is often paroxysmal. Each episode starts and ends abruptly, lasting seconds to minutes, and may recur frequently (> 5–6 times per day)
- Paroxysmal pruritus can be successfully treated by anti-epileptic drugs such as carbamazepine, phenytoin, or gabapentin. However, electroencephalographic (EEG) studies do not support an epileptic mechanism in the cortex for central neurogenic pruritus
- The location of pruritus may be segmental or dermatomal
- The attacks of pruritus can awake the patient from sleep and may cause insomnia
- Paroxysmal pruritus may be accompanied by paroxysmal or constant pain (burning and aching) in the same area (pruralgia)

activity that may sensitize the second-order neuron in the spinal cord and supraspinal centres may be sensitized. In an early stage, damage to the peripheral fibres induces axonal degeneration (slow Wallerian degeneration).[3] This process is still poorly understood, but is crucial to the next phase: regeneration. Both degeneration and regeneration may depend on specific genes[4] and may differ from patient to patient. After nerve damage, regeneration may be incomplete and/or aberrant, and pruritus may occur. Some patients with intractable pruritus due to neuropathy have a history of atopic dermatitis in childhood. Most patients with intractable pruritus caused by neuropathy have incomplete and/or aberrant regenerated fibres that are much more sensitive to pruritogens. Constant afferent input causes spinal sensitization that may sometimes be irreversible (see Chapter 2).

Peripheral neuropathy may cause anaesthesia, hypaesthesia, hyperalgesia, and allodynia. These symptoms are more often encountered than alloknesis or hyperknesis. The reason for this symptom complex is that most of the C-fibres that are damaged are pain-transmitting fibres—only about 5% of all C-fibres specifically mediate pruritus.[2, 5] Interestingly, pain elicited by damage to pain-specific C-fibres may inhibit pruritus.[6] This is true for normal subjects. There is some evidence that suggests a central sensitization for pruritus in patients with chronic pruritus. Such patients may perceive pain as pruritus.

Most, if not all, factors that damage unmyelinated C-fibres are not specific to pruritus fibres. To produce persistent pruritus, specific and selective impulses need to stimulate the pruritus-transmitting second-order neurons in the spinal cord, without concomitant activation of the inhibiting interneurons. Additionally, this specific pruritic input can sensitize the spinal cord, such that originally noxious stimuli can be perceived as pruritus. A population of second-order pruritus neurons in the spinothalamic tract, specifically excited by iontophoretically administered histamine, has been identified in the dorsal horn.[7] Disinhibition of this mechanism in the spinal cord by, for example, opioid analgesics, may result in pruritus (see Chapter 7).

Herpes zoster

Herpes zoster infection may cause postherpetic neuralgia, but occasionally it may be responsible for postherpetic pruritus.[8, 9] After recovery from herpetic infection, skin innervation may remain diminished.[9] Loss of skin innervation caused by neuronal damage may be compensated by regeneration of damaged fibres or 'collateral sprouting' of adjacent undamaged nerves. Damaged nerves respond to increased activity of nerve growth factors (NGFs).[10]

Abnormal sprouting, probably due to increased activity of the NGFs, occurs not only in and around the peripheral sites of damage, but also occurs in the dorsal horn of the spinal cord.[11] This process may be responsible for sensitization to input from the A-β tactile fibres[12] and may cause hyperpathia and allodynia. Occasionally, as a result of regeneration of the pruritus-specific C-fibres, the same process may result in hyperknesis and alloknesis. Regenerated fibres may be extremely sensitive to histamine (or may be spontaneously active without any stimulation). These phenomena constitute the basis of sensitization of the spinal cord, which frequently adds a central and poorly reversible process to peripheral nerve damage.

Senile pruritus

Many old people experience 'senile pruritus'. It has been suggested that senile pruritus may be related to peripheral nerve injury in ageing skin, that it may be analogous in some respects to phantom limb pain.[13] Indeed, loss of neurons in ageing skin is probably responsible for impaired thermal regulation, reduced tactile sensitivity, and impaired pain perception.[14] Concomitant loss of nociceptive neurons in the skin could also be responsible for pruritus, as a result of reduced neural inhibition. Recently, amelioration of senile pruritus associated with administration of cyclosporin A[15] or thalidomide[16] has been described. These observations suggest that senile pruritus is not only attributable to dry, atrophic skin. It seems probable that senile pruritus results from immunological damage to the basement membrane of the skin and nerves.[17]

Itchy scars

Regenerating sprouts originating from damaged axons are frequently hypersensitive to histamine.[10, 18] In early wounds increased levels of histamine, serotonin, bradykinin, and prostaglandins have been found.[19, 20] Pruritus usually subsides as the scar matures. In some instances, especially in keloid scars, pruritus may persist for months or years. Similar phenomena may also apply to anal fissures.[21] Aberrant regeneration and sprouting may result in the formation of peripheral itchy neuromas.[22] Intralesional corticosteroids or doxepin 5% cream may be used for the treatment of the early itchy scars.[23]

Amyloidosis

Primary amyloidosis is frequently associated with severe, intractable pruritus.[24–26] In the lichenified parts of the skin of otherwise healthy individuals, secondary accumulation of amyloid is frequently found.[27] Patches of amyloid may be responsible for pruritus by an unknown mechanism.

Diabetes mellitus

Diabetes is rarely if ever associated with a pruritic neuropathy. However, the incidences of diabetes mellitus and peripheral neuropathy are both relatively high. Therefore occasional reports of the coexistence between neuropathy and pruritus are insufficient to establish a causal relationship.[28–30] In one series of 100 diabetic patients, generalized pruritus was reported in only 8 patients. This frequency is not significantly greater than the corresponding frequency in non-diabetic patients.[29] However, other types of pruritus are common in diabetic patients. For example, pruritus in these patients may be associated with poor diabetic control and fungal growth on skin and mucous membranes (e.g. the vulva).[31]

Drug-induced neuropathy

Several drugs can cause neuropathy. Some of these neuropathies are known to be associated with pruritus (see Chapter 8). Drug-induced neuropathies, not discussed elsewhere in this book, are presented briefly here.

Hydroxyethyl starch

Hydroxyethyl starch (HES) is used in the treatment of various cochleovestibular disorders, such as sudden hearing loss, neuronopathia vestibularis, and idiopathic facial palsy. It improves the microcirculation better than the previously used dextran. In one study of 149 patients treated with HES, nearly 30% complained of pruritus lasting from 6 weeks to 6 months.[32] The pruritus was resistant to H_1-antihistamines. In a second trial the incidence of pruritus was only 10%.[33] The occurrence of pruritus is dose-dependent.[34] Patients with persistent pruritus consistently have deposition of HES in small peripheral nerves. HES-reactive vacuoles have been demonstrated in the Schwann cells of both unmyelinated and small myelinated nerve fibres, and in endoneural and perineural cells. Neural devacuolization paralleled improvement in pruritus.[35, 36] Severe pruritus caused by HES therapy has been successfully treated with capsaicin.[37] Opioid antagonists are also helpful.[38]

Gold and other heavy metals

Gold salts are widely used in the treatment of rheumatoid arthritis. Their use is sometimes associated with neuropathy and pruritus.[39–41] In some cases gold may be the cause of severe neurological impairment and disability.[41] Some of the changes may start with a dermatosis, but pruritus may persist after disappearance of the rash. Smokers and HLA Bw35 positive patients, and perhaps atopic patients, are more prone to gold drug reaction.[39, 41] Gold salts may also cause liver toxicity and insufficiency, which may also be a cause of pruritus.[42] Discontinuation of the gold salt alone may lead to recovery. In severe neuropathy, dimercaprol may be used.[43, 44] However, this drug is not included in several European formularies.

Various other heavy metals may be neurotoxic and cause pruritus. One of them is mercury, which is used in dentistry.[45] Two patients, seen by the author because of generalized intractable pruritus, had multiple dental fillings; a change to non-mercurial fillings led to a resolution of the pruritus. It is not known if other heavy metals can be responsible for neuropathy and pruritus. Cisplatin and carboplatin, which are widely used in oncology, may cause neuropathy, although there are no reports of these agents inducing neuropathic pruritus.

Nerve entrapment

Another form of neural damage, usually less permanent, is nerve compression or nerve entrapment. In this context, as said before, pruritus is usually only one of many symptoms because the neuropathy affects whole nerves. Nerves include afferent and efferent fibres of many kinds. There are several syndromes associated with nerve entrapment (Table 10.2). Notalgia paraesthetica, the typical and most common syndrome of nerve entrapment, will be highlighted.

Notalgia paraesthetica

This nerve entrapment syndrome is associated with paraesthesias and pruritus. It was first described by Astwazaturow in 1934.[46] Later this syndrome was described many times under different names. A hereditary

Table 10.2 Nerve entrapment syndromes that may be complicated by paraesthesia and pruritus

Syndrome	Nerve involved	References
Brachioradial pruritus	Cutaneous branch of radial nerve	61, 85, 86
Notalgia paraesthetica	Entrapment or denervation of T_{2-6} dorsal root ganglions	87–90
Meralgia paresthetica	Lateral femoral cutaneous nerve	91–96
Cheiralgia paresthetica	Radial nerve	97–99
Carpal tunnel syndrome	Median nerve	100
Cervical rib syndrome	Brachial plexus	101
Gonyalgia paraesthetica	Saphenous nerve	102

syndrome of notalgia paraesthetica associated with medullary thyroid carcinoma[47] and multiple endocrine neoplasia type 2A has been described.[25, 48–50] Thus, this syndrome may be regarded as a paraneoplastic one (see Chapter 8).

The syndrome involves intense pruritus of the back, between the scapulae. Intensive rubbing and scratching may lead to lichenification of the skin and an increase in the density of skin innervation.[51] Notalgia paraesthetica responds well to administration of capsaicin cream 0.025%.[52–54] Capsaicin is known to cause skin C-fibre atrophy (see Chapter 12).[55] In notalgia paraesthetica increased dermal innervation has been found,[51] probably secondary to scratching and rubbing,[55–57] and it is possible that capsaicin disrupts the vicious cycle of pruritus–scratching–inflammation–increased intradermal innervation–lichenification/amyloid deposition–pruritus.

Pruritus caused by spinal or supraspinal injury

Besides pruritus secondary to peripheral nerve damage, occasionally patients experience severe pruritus after brain or spinal cord damage,[58] for example, in association with a tumour,[59–61] stroke,[62–64] aneurysm,[65] or abscess.[66, 67] In these situations the pruritus may be uni- or bilateral, with or without involvement of the homologous side of the face. As is usual with brain disorders, the pruritus is experienced on the side contralateral to the lesion. Severe paroxysmal pruritus caused by cerebral lesions has occurred in patients with multiple sclerosis.[68–73] Finally, spinal tumours with focal damage may also cause severe pruritus.[60, 61, 74]

Therapy: general considerations

Neuropathic pruritus often responds to treatments similar to those used for painful neuropathies. Tricyclic antidepressants may be useful.[75–77] Doxepin is probably the first choice (see Chapter 13).[78, 79] However, no definitive studies have been published. Also, a 5% doxepin topical cream may be useful.[23, 80, 81] Paroxysmal pruritus in multiple sclerosis and patients with other central lesions is best treated with anti-epileptic drugs. Carbamazepine and phenytoin have been used in this context for many years. However, gabapentin is better tolerated by most patients and does not induce liver enzymes and thereby change the pharmacology of many other drugs and endogenous substrates. In some patients, nonsteroidal anti-inflammatory drugs (NSAIDs), by inhibiting prostaglandin synthesis, may desensitize peripheral nerve endings and decrease itching.[82, 83]

Capsaicin often appears to be effective in notalgia paraesthetica,[53, 54, 84] and may be tried in other nerve entrapment syndromes.

Conclusions

* Pruritus may be a consequence of nerve damage or entrapment.
* Neuropathy complicated by pruritus is rare.
* Some drugs, such as hydroxyethyl starch and gold salts, induce pruritus but not pain.
* Nerve entrapment causes diverse localized pruritus syndromes that may be unrecognized but present for many years.
* Treatment of pruritic neuropathy is similar to that of painful neuropathy. This implies that our arsenal of effective drugs is limited.

References

1. Twycross R, Greaves MW, Handwerker H, *et al.* (2003). Itch: scratching more than the surface. *Q JM* **96**:7–26.
2. Schmidt R, Schmelz M, Ringkamp M, Handwerker HO, Torebjörk HE. (1997). Innervation territories of mechanically activated C nociceptor units in human skin. *J Neurophysiol* **78**:2641–8.
3. Ramer MS, French GD, Bisby MA. (1997). Wallerian degeneration is required for both neuropathic pain and sympathetic sprouting into the DRG. *Pain* **72**:71–8.
4. Wang M, Wu Y, Culver DG, Glass JD. (2001). The gene for slow Wallerian degeneration (Wld(s)) is also protective against vincristine neuropathy. *Neurobiol Dis* **8**:155–61.
5. Schmelz M, Schmidt R, Bickel A, Handwerker HO, Torebjörk HE. (1997). Specific C-receptors for itch in human skin. *J Neurosci* **17**:8003–8.
6. Greaves MW, Wall PD. (1996). Pathophysiology of itching. *Lancet* **348**:938–40.
7. Andrew D, Craig AD. (2001). Spinothalamic lamina I neurons selectively sensitive to histamine: a central neural pathway for itch. *Nat Neurosci* **4**:72–7.
8. Liddell K. (1974). Post-herpetic pruritus. *Br Med J* **4**:165.
9. Oaklander AL, Cohen SP, Raju SV. (2002). Intractable postherpetic itch and cutaneous deafferentation after facial shingles. *Pain* **96**:9–12.
10. Inbal R, Rousso M, Ashur H, Wall PD, Devor M. (1987). Collateral sprouting in skin and sensory recovery after nerve injury in man. *Pain* **28**:141–54.
11. Romero MI, Rangappa N, Li L, Lightfoot E, Garry MG, Smith GM. (2000). Extensive sprouting of sensory afferents and hyperalgesia induced by conditional expression of nerve growth factor in the adult spinal cord. *J Neurosci* **20**:4435–45.

12. Baron R, Saguer M. (1993). Postherpetic neuralgia. Are C-nociceptors involved in signalling and maintenance of tactile allodynia? *Brain* **116**(Pt. 6):1477–96.

13. Bernhard JD. (1992). Phantom itch, pseudophantom itch, and senile pruritus. *Int J Dermatol* **31**:856–7.

14. Balin AK, Pratt LA. (1989). Physiological consequences of human skin aging. *Cutis* **43**:431–6.

15. Teofoli P, De Pita O, Frezzolini A, Lotti T. (1998). Antipruritic effect of oral cyclosporin A in essential senile pruritus. *Acta Derm Venereol* **78**:232.

16. Daly BM, Shuster S. (2000). Antipruritic action of thalidomide. *Acta Derm Venereol* **80**:24–5.

17. Bernhard JD. (1997). Do anti-basement membrane zone antibodies cause some cases of 'senile pruritus'? *Arch Dermatol* **133**:1049–50.

18. Simone DA, Alreja M, LaMotte RH. (1991). Psychophysical studies of the itch sensation and itchy skin ('alloknesis') produced by intracutaneous injection of histamine. *Somatosens Mot Res* **8**:271–9.

19. Cohen IK, Beaven MA, Horakova Z, Keiser HR. (1972). Histamine and collagen synthesis in keloid and hypertrophic scar. *Surg Forum* **23**:509–10.

20. Nara T. (1985). Histamine and 5-hydroxytryptamine in human scar tissue. *Ann Plast Surg* **14**:244–7.

21. Horsch D, Kirsch JJ, Weihe E. (1998). Elevated density and plasticity of nerve fibres in anal fissures. *Int J Colorectal Dis* **13**:134–40.

22. Cramer HJ, Heerwagen E. (1980). Chronic vulvar pruritus caused by terminal-fibre neuroma episiotomy scar. *Zentralbl Gynakol* **102**:1437–43.

23. Drake LA, Fallon JD, Sober A. (1994). Relief of pruritus in patients with atopic dermatitis after treatment with topical doxepin cream. The Doxepin Study Group. *J Am Acad Dermatol* **31**:613–6.

24. Newton JA, Jagjivan A, Bhogal B, McKee PH, McGibbon DH. (1985). Familial primary cutaneous amyloidosis. *Br J Dermatol* **112**:201–8.

25. Ferrer JP, Halperin I, Conget JI, *et al.* (1991). Primary localized cutaneous amyloidosis and familial medullary thyroid carcinoma. *Clin Endocrinol (Oxf)* **34**:435–9.

26. Simon A, Dode C, van der Meer JW, Drenth JP. (2001). Familial periodic fever and amyloidosis due to a new mutation in the TNFRSF1A gene. *Am J Med* **110**:313–16.

27. Pena-Penabad MC, Garcia-Silva J, Armijo M. (1995). Notalgia paraesthetica and macular amyloidosis: cause–effect relationship? *Clin Exp Dermatol* **20**:279.

28. Scribner M. (1977). Diabetes and pruritus of the scalp. *J Am Med Assoc* **237**:1559.

29. Neilly JB, Martin A, Simpson N, MacCuish AC. (1986). Pruritus in diabetes mellitus: investigation of prevalence and correlation with diabetes control. *Diabetes Care* **9**:273–5.

30. Schwartz J, Rosenfeld V. (1993). Clonidine for painful diabetic–uremic leg cramps and pruritus—a case report. *Angiology* **44**:985.

31. Kantor GR, Lookingbill DP. (1983). Generalized pruritus and systemic disease. *J Am Acad Dermatol* **9**:375–82.

32. Kakigi R. (1994). Diffuse noxious inhibitory control. Reappraisal by pain-related somatosensory evoked potentials following CO_2 laser stimulation. *J Neurol Sci* **125**:198–205.

33. Bothner U, Georgieff M, Vogt NH. (1998). Assessment of the safety and tolerance of 6% hydroxyethyl starch (200/0.5) solution: a randomized, controlled epidemiology study. *Anesth Analg* **86**:850–5.

34. Kimme P, Jannsen B, Ledin T, Gupta A, Vegfors M. (2001). High incidence of pruritus after large doses of hydroxyethyl starch (HES) infusions. *Acta Anaesthesiol Scand* **45**:686–9.

35. Metze D, Reimann S, Szepfalusi Z, Bohle B, Kraft D, Luger TA. (1997). Persistent pruritus after hydroxyethyl starch infusion therapy: a result of long-term storage in cutaneous nerves. *Br J Dermatol* **136**:553–9.

36. Sirtl C, Laubenthal H, Zumtobel V, Kraft D, Jurecka W. (1999). Tissue deposits of hydroxyethyl starch (HES): dose-dependent and time-related. *Br J Anaesth* **82**:510–5.

37. Szeimies RM, Stolz W, Wlotzke U, Korting HC, Landthaler M. (1994). Successful treatment of hydroxyethyl starch-induced pruritus with topical capsaicin. *Br J Dermatol* **131**:380–2.

38. Metze D, Reimann S, Beissert S, Luger T. (1999). Efficacy and safety of naltrexone, an oral opiate receptor antagonist, in the treatment of pruritus in internal and dermatological diseases. *J Am Acad Dermatol* **41**:533–9.

39. Bonnetblanc JM. (1996). Cutaneous reactions to gold salts. *Presse Med* **25**:1555–8.

40. Russell MA, Langley M, Truett AP 3rd, King LE Jr, Boyd AS. (1997). Lichenoid dermatitis after consumption of gold-containing liquor. *J Am Acad Dermatol* **36**:841–4.

41. Fam AG, Gordon DA, Sarkozi J, *et al.* (1984). Neurologic complications associated with gold therapy for rheumatoid arthritis. *J Rheumatol* **11**:700–6.

42. Fleischner GM, Morecki R, Hanaichi T, Hayashi H, Quintana N, Sternlieb I. (1991). Light- and electron-microscopical study of a case of gold salt-induced hepatotoxicity. *Hepatology* **14**:422–5.

43. England JM, Smith DS. (1972). Gold-induced thrombocytopenia and response to dimercaprol. *Br Med J* **2**:748–9.

44. Hughes RD, Gazzard BG, Murray-Lyon IM, Williams RS. (1976). The use of cysteamine and dimercaprol. *J Int Med Res* **4**:123–9.

45. Forsell M, Marcusson JA, Carlmark B, Johansson O. (1997). Analysis of the metal content of *in vivo*-fixed dental alloys by means of a simple office procedure. *Swed Dent J* **21**:161–8.

46. Astwazaturow M. (1934). Der paresthetische Neuralgien und einde bezondere Form derselben—Nothalgia paresthetica. *Nervenarzt* **133**:88.

47. Nunziata V, Giannattasio R, Di Giovanni G, D'Armiento MR, Mancini M. (1989). Hereditary localized pruritus in affected members of a kindred with multiple endocrine neoplasia type 2A (Sipple's syndrome). *Clin Endocrinol (Oxf)* **30**:57–63.

48. Gagel RF, Levy ML, Donovan DT, Alford BR, Wheeler T, Tschen JA. (1989). Multiple endocrine neoplasia type 2a associated with cutaneous lichen amyloidosis. *Ann Intern Med* **111**:802–6.

49. Bugalho MJ, Limbert E, Sobrinho LG, *et al.* (1992). A kindred with multiple endocrine neoplasia type 2A associated with pruritic skin lesions. *Cancer* **70**:2664–7.

50. Rivollier C, Emy P, Armingaud P, *et al.* (1999). Paresthetic notalgia and multiple endocrine neoplasia type 2a (Sipple's syndrome): 3 cases. *Ann Dermatol Venereol* **126**:522–4.

51. Springall DR, Karanth SS, Kirkham N, Darley CR, Polak JM. (1991). Symptoms of notalgia paresthetica may be explained by increased dermal innervation. *J Invest Dermatol* **97**:555–61.

52. Wallengren J. (1991). Treatment of notalgia paresthetica with topical capsaicin. *J Am Acad Dermatol* **24**:286–8.

53. Leibsohn E. (1992). Treatment of notalgia paresthetica with capsaicin. *Cutis* **49**:335–6.

54. Wallengren J, Klinker M. (1995). Successful treatment of notalgia paresthetica with topical capsaicin: vehicle-controlled, double-blind, crossover study. *J Am Acad Dermatol* **32**:287–9.

55. Dux M, Sann H, Schemann M, Jancso G. (1999). Changes in fibre populations of the rat hairy skin following selective chemodenervation by capsaicin. *Cell Tissue Res* **296**:471–7.

56. Wong CK, Lin CS. (1988). Friction amyloidosis. *Int J Dermatol* **27**:302–7.

57. Sumitra S, Yesudian P. (1993). Friction amyloidosis: a variant or an etiologic factor in amyloidosis cutis? *Int J Dermatol* **32**:422–3.

58. Canavero S, Bonicalzi V, Massa-Micon B. (1997). Central neurogenic pruritus: a literature review. *Acta Neurol Belg* **97**:244–7.

59. Andreev VC, Petkov I. (1975). Skin manifestations associated with tumours of the brain. *Br J Dermatol* **92**:675–8.

60. Johnson RE, Kanigsberg ND, Jimenez CL. (2000). Localized pruritus: a presenting symptom of a spinal cord tumor in a child with features of neurofibromatosis. *J Am Acad Dermatol* **43**:958–61.

61. Kavak A, Dosoglu M. (2002). Can a spinal cord tumor cause brachioradial pruritus? *J Am Acad Dermatol* **46**:437–40.

62. Massey EW. (1984). Unilateral neurogenic pruritus following stroke. *Stroke* **15**:901–3.

63. Shapiro PE, Braun CW. (1987). Unilateral pruritus after a stroke. *Arch Dermatol* **123**:1527–30.

64. Kimyai-Asadi A, Nousari HC, Kimyai-Asadi T, Milani F. (1999). Poststroke pruritus. *Stroke* **30**:692–3.

65. Vuadens P, Regli F, Dolivo M, Uske A. (1994). Segmental pruritus and intramedullary vascular malformation. *Schweiz Arch Neurol Psychiatr* **145**:13–6.

66. Sullivan MJ, Drake ME Jr. (1984). Unilateral pruritus and Nocardia brain abscess. *Neurology* **34**:828–9.

67. Weintraub E, Robinson C, Newmeyer M. (2000). Catastrophic medical complication in psychogenic excoriation. *South Med J* **93**:1099–101.

68. Osterman PO. (1976). Paroxysmal itching in multiple sclerosis. *Br J Dermatol* **95**:555–8.

69. Yabuki S, Hayabara T. (1979). Paroxysmal dysesthesia in multiple sclerosis. *Folia Psychiatr Neurol Jpn* **33**:97–104.

70. Osterman PO. (1979). Paroxysmal itching in multiple sclerosis. *Int J Dermatol* **18**:626–7.

71. Yamamoto M, Yabuki S, Hayabara T, Otsuki S. (1981). Paroxysmal itching in multiple sclerosis: a report of three cases. *J Neurol Neurosurg Psychiatry* **44**:19–22.

72. Sandyk R. (1994). Paroxysmal itching in multiple sclerosis during treatment with external magnetic fields. *Int J Neurosci* **75**:65–71.

73. Taylor RS. (1998). Multiple sclerosis potpourri. Paroxysmal symptoms, seizures, fatigue, pregnancy, and more. *Phys Med Rehabil Clin N Am* **9**:551–9.

74. Kinsella LJ, Carney-Godley K, Feldmann E. (1992). Lichen simplex chronicus as the initial manifestation of intramedullary neoplasm and syringomyelia. *Neurosurgery* **30**:418–21.

75. Figge J, Leonard P, Richelson E. (1979). Tricyclic antidepressants: potent blockade of histamine H1 receptors of guinea pig ileum. *Eur J Pharmacol* **58**:479–83.

76. Richelson E. (1983). Antimuscarinic and other receptor-blocking properties of antidepressants. *Mayo Clin Proc* **58**:40–6.

77. Groene D, Martus P, Heyer G. (2001). Doxepin affects acetylcholine induced cutaneous reactions in atopic eczema. *Exp Dermatol* **10**:110–17.

78. Figueiredo A, Ribeiro CA, Goncalo M, Almeida L, Poiares-Baptista A, Teixeira F. (1990). Mechanism of action of doxepin in the treatment of chronic urticaria. *Fundam Clin Pharmacol* **4**:147–58.

79. Smith PF, Corelli RL. (1997). Doxepin in the management of pruritus associated with allergic cutaneous reactions. *Ann Pharmacother* **31**:633–5.

80. Breneman D, Dunlap F, Monroe E. (1997). Doxepin cream relieves eczema-associated pruritus within 15 minutes and is not accompanied by a risk of rebound upon discontinuation. *J Dermatol Treatm* **8**:161–8.

81. Anonymous. (2000). Doxepin cream for eczema? *Drug Ther Bull* **38**:31–2.

82. Khan OA. (1994). Treatment of paroxysmal symptoms in multiple sclerosis with ibuprofen. *Neurology* **44**:571–2.

83. Smith KJ, Skelton HG, Yeager J, Lee RB, Wagner KF. (1997). Pruritus in HIV-1 disease: therapy with drugs which may modulate the pattern of immune dysregulation. *Dermatology* **195**:353–8.

84. Raison-Peyron N, Meunier L, Acevedo M, Meynadier J. (1999). Notalgia paresthetica: clinical, physiopathological and therapeutic aspects. A study of 12 cases. *J Eur Acad Dermatol Venereol* **12**:215–21.

85. Weintraub E, Robinson C, Newmeyer M. (2000). Catastrophic medical complication in psychogenic excoriation. *South Med J* **93**:1099–101.

86. Osterman PO. (1976). Paroxysmal itching in multiple sclerosis. *Br J Dermatol* **95**:555–8.

87. Yabuki S, Hayabara T. (1979). Paroxysmal dyseshesia in multiple sclerosis. *Folia Psychiatr Neurol Jpn* **33**:97–104.

88. Osterman PO. (1979). Paroxysmal itching in multiple sclerosis. *Int J Dermatol* **18**:626–7.

89. Yamamoto M, Yabuki S, Hayabara T, Otsuki S. (1981). Paroxysmal itching in multiple sclerosis: a report of three cases. *J Neurol Neurosurg Psychiatry* **44**:19–22.

90. Sandyk R. (1994). Paroxysmal itching in multiple sclerosis during treatment with external magnetic fields. *Int J Neurosci* **75**:65–71.

91. Taylor RS. (1998). Multiple sclerosis potpourri. Paroxysmal symptoms, seizures, fatigue, pregnancy, and more. *Phys Med Rehabil Clin N Am* **9**:551–9.

92. Kinsella LJ, Carney-Godley K, Feldmann E. (1992). Lichen simplex chronicus as the initial manifestation of intramedullary neoplasm and syringomyelia. *Neurosurgery* **30**:418–21.

93. Figge J, Leonard P, Richelson E. (1979). Tricyclic antidepressants: potent blockade of histamine H1 receptors of guinea pig ileum. *Eur J Pharmacol* **58**:479–83.

94. Richelson E. (1983). Antimuscarinic and other receptor-blocking properties of antidepressants. *Mayo Clin Proc* **58**:40–6.

95. Groene D, Martus P, Heyer G. (2001). Doxepin affects acetylcholine induced cutaneous reactions in atopic eczema. *Exp Dermatol* **10**:110–7.

96. Figueiredo A, Ribeiro CA, Goncalo M, Almeida L, Poiares-Baptista A, Teixeira F. (1990). Mechanism of action of doxepin in the treatment of chronic urticaria. *Fundam Clin Pharmacol* **4**:147–58.

97. Smith PF, Corelli RL. (1997). Doxepin in the management of pruritus associated with allergic cutaneous reactions. *Ann Pharmacother* **31**:633–5.

98. Breneman D, Dunlap E, Monroe E. (1997). *J Dermatol Treatm.* **8**:161–8(Abstr.).

99. Anonymous. (2000). Doxepin cream for eczema? *Drug Ther Bull* **38**:31–2.

100. Khan OA. (1994). Treatment of paroxysmal symptoms in multiple sclerosis with ibuprofen. *Neurology* **44**:571–2.

101. Smith KJ, Skelton HG, Yeager J, Lee RB, Wagner KF. (1997). Pruritus in HIV-1 disease: therapy with drugs which may modulate the pattern of immune dysregulation. *Dermatology* **195**:353–8.

102. Raison-Peyron N, Meunier L, Acevedo M, Meynadier J. (1999). Notalgia paresthetica: clinical, physiopathological and therapeutic aspects. A study of 12 cases. *J Eur Acad Dermatol Venereol* **12**:215–21.

11

Psychogenic pruritus

John Y. Koo and Roger S. Lo

Psychogenic pruritus: a diagnosis of exclusion?

Apart from making a psychiatric referral, which the patient may not accept, most dermatologists are often not clear about how to proceed beyond concluding that pruritus without primary skin lesions and evidence of underlying organic disease must be psychogenic in origin. In this chapter we shall address several questions about this phenomenon.

- What positive findings can be expected in psychogenic pruritus?

- How would one distinguish between psychogenic and neurogenic pruritus?

- What are the differential diagnoses falling under the umbrella term 'psychogenic pruritus'?

- What are the therapeutic options available to all of us?

- Is it appropriate to use psychotropic medications?

Psychogenic pruritus should not be considered as simply a diagnosis of exclusion. In fact, it encompasses a heterogeneous group of diagnoses based on distinct clinical phenomena and pathophysiological mechanisms requiring different diagnostic and therapeutic strategies. Misdiagnosis of psychogenic pruritus can have serious consequences, as it did for one patient with an epidural abscess who developed paraplegia.[1] Further, the presence of primary skin lesions does not necessarily exclude a psychogenic component. Studies have shown that psychological factors modulate the perception of pruritus in many skin disorders including psoriasis, atopic dermatitis, and lichen simplex chronicus. These conditions have been termed as 'psychophysiological', meaning skin disorder exacerbated by factors such as psychological stress.[2] In these cases, the patients may derive much benefit from having their underlying psychological disorders correctly diagnosed and treated.

Definition and classification

Psychogenic pruritus can be viewed as falling into two categories. The first of them is pruritus precipitated and/or created by conscious behavioural response to underlying psychopathology. In these cases, itchy lesions are entirely secondary to manipulation of normal skin. This category includes:

- pruritus secondary to picking and formication in a conscious response to the demands of a delusional belief (i.e. monosymptomatic hypochondriacal psychosis).

- pruritus initiated by and secondary to conscious repetitive actions such as picking, scratching, or rubbing driven by obsession and compulsion (neurotic excoriation, acne, and excoriée). Two main forms of primary neurotic excoriation exist: patients who pick and scratch from itching; or patients who pick and scratch from a desire to remove a benign skin lesion. About 10% of patients have never experienced a primary itch.[3]

- Itchy lesions produced consciously for a secondary gain that is consciously calculated (i.e. malingering).

The second category is pruritus initiated through unconscious pathological mental processing. This includes pruritus as an indirect manifestation of depression and/or anxiety and represents repressed psychological conflicts. The term hallucinatory pruritus has also been used and this type of psychogenic pruritus can be accompanied by a variety of hallucinatory tactile sensations such as burning, aching, and stinging.

Phenomenology of psychogenic pruritus

Phenomenology is the psychiatric equivalent of the term morphology used in dermatology. Unlike skin lesions, most mental deviations cannot be directly and conveniently visualized—hence the use of the term phenomenology rather than morphology.

Besides the absence of primary skin lesions, certain clinical findings suggest that the psychogenic pruritus can be CNS-mediated including neurogenic. Frequently, pruritus is associated with an observable psychiatric problem, especially anxiety and/or depression, but occasionally obsessive–compulsive disorder and psychosis with delusional ideations. In this context, a chronological association, where the onset of psychological stress or disorder precedes the onset of pruritus, can be suggestive of psychogenic pruritus. However, it is often very difficult to ascertain whether the observed psychopathology (such as anxiety or depression) is primary or secondary to the pruritus. On the other hand, this distinction is not as critical as it may seem because it is well established that secondary psychopathologies can enhance pruritus perception. Therefore, an associated psychopathology should be treated whether or not it is thought to be primary or secondary to the pruritus. In fact, in cases where the temporal relationship between the onset of psychopathology and pruritus is difficult to ascertain, it is better to ignore the question about whether pruritus is primary or secondary to psychopathology.

At times, when the patient has insight into his/her condition, the clinical clue comes directly from the patient. For instance, patients with neurotic excoriation, which is associated with obsessive–compulsive disorder (OCD), may acknowledge the self-inflicted nature of the excoriated lesions, leading to a cycle of itch–compulsive scratch–itch.[4]

Another important clue to the possible psychogenic origin of pruritus comes from its paroxysmal nature. Paroxysmal pruritus is usually intense with sudden onset and sudden resolution, with no pruritus in between the episodes. However, paroxysmal pruritus can be either neurogenic (see Chapter 10) or psychogenic, and it is important to try to distinguish between the two. Although rare in the literature (for reviews see references 5 and 6), pruritus can present as the dominant symptom of a central or peripheral nervous system lesion (see Chapter 10). These neuropathic causes occur in the absence of primary skin lesions and should be considered in the differential diagnoses of psychogenic pruritus (see also Fig. 10.1). The prominent characteristics of neuropathic pruritus, which can be helpful in distinguishing neuropathic from psychogenic pruritus, are outlined in the previous chapter (see Box 10.1)

Moreover, obvious pleasure associated with the itch and scratch cycle hints at a psychogenic origin. In psychoanalytic terms, this process of somatization is referred to as autoerotic pruritus where physical symptoms are regarded as an expression of the unconscious sexual drive. This pleasure-deriving itch–scratch cycle may be especially evident in cases of neuro-dermatitis (lichen simplex chronicus).

Should psychogenic pruritus cease during sleep?

According to the conventional wisdom, psychogenic pruritus should cease during sleep, while organic pruritus can awaken the patient at night. This may relate to the generalization that organic pruritus is simply more severe or to a possible differential interaction of psychogenic and organic pruritus with sleep-related CNS factors. On the other hand Gupta et al.[7] concluded that psychiatric factors (e.g. depression) underlying an itchy dermatosis (e.g. psoriasis) determine awakening from sleep. This suggests that arousal from sleep in association with pruritus is not always because of increased afferent sensory input from the skin. In other words, the CNS may play a role in the initiation and modulation of pruritus perception. However, because Gupta et al. studied only patients with primary skin disease with underlying psychopathologies, their findings cannot be extrapolated to all patients with generalized pruritus without a primary skin disease.[8] In other words, a psychogenic cause cannot be ruled out automatically just because the pruritus is associated with nocturnal wakening.

Pathogenesis of psychogenic pruritus

Neither psychogenic nor organic pruritus exists in a pure form. Pruritus with a psychogenic origin can result in anatomical and neurochemical changes that perpetuate and maintain the symptom.[9] Psychosomatic and individual coping strategies have been shown to be predictors of skin responsiveness to experimentally (histamine-) induced pruritus in humans.[10]

At the molecular level, the bidirectional loop between the CNS and peripheral pruritogenic processes has been well appreciated as it relates to stress.[11] For instance, cutaneous neuropeptides are contained in myelinated A-δ fibres and small unmyelinated C-fibres, including sensory and autonomic fibres (see Chapter 2). The skin is innervated not only by primary afferent sensory nerves but also by post-ganglionic cholinergic parasympathetic and adrenergic and cholinergic sympathetic nerves. The former not only serve to conduct stimuli from the skin to the CNS but also act in an efferent 'neurosecretory' manner. Thus, emotional stress-induced release of neuropeptides can be pruritogenic and can also act on the immune system via humoral factors such as cytokines and antibodies. This in turn regulates neuroendocrine function. The neuropeptides also exert their multiple effects on central regulatory centres that can in turn regulate autonomic and behavioural responses.

With regard to psychopathology, it has been proposed that the depressed clinical state, which has been shown to be associated with elevated levels of corticotropin-releasing hormone (CRH), amplifies pruritus perception by increasing central nervous endogenous opioid levels.[12] This hypothesis highlights the recent finding of psychoneuroimmunological links. For example, acute immobilization stress triggers skin mast cell degranulation via CRH, neurotensin (NT), and substance P (SP) in rats.[13] Thus, stress and depression may share a common mediator of pruritus, namely, CRH.

Stress and pruritus

That a relationship between stress and pruritus may exist centrally is further supported by the findings that unpredictable and stressful conditions may activate the opioid pathway, enhancing pruritus sensation.[14] Peripherally, histamine, vasoactive neuropeptides, and mediators of inflammation may also be liberated by emotional stress, while stress-related haemodynamic changes, variations in skin temperature, and the sweat response all may contribute to existing pruritus. Scratching, a common behavioural response to stress, may compound the problem through initiating an itch–scratch–itch cycle. Further, one cannot ignore observation that the pruritus threshold varies with respect to emotional stress or the time of day. There appears to be a lower pruritus threshold at night as compared to the daytime, and this may relate to the possible lowering of pruritus threshold when the patient is not busy with or distracted by a hectic daytime schedule.[15, 16]

Depression and pruritus

Similarly, studies have shown that depression can enhance pruritus perception. Several reports by Gupta *et al.* showed that depression modulates pruritus perception in psychophysiological disorders such as psoriasis, atopic dermatitis, and chronic idiopathic urticaria.[12, 17–19] According to these authors there was a positive statistically significant correlation between pruritus severity and severity of depressive symptoms.

The pathogenesis of psychogenic pruritus can also be viewed from a psychodynamic or psychoanalytic point of view. Here, the skin is a channel for expression of traumatic early experiences or difficult, unconscious, and unresolved psychological conflict(s). That is, pruritus represents a somatic symptom of repressed intrapsychic conflict. Many case reports and uncontrolled studies of successful psychotherapy for intractable psychogenic pruritus suggest the validity of this more psychologically comprehensive view of disease.[20]

Differential diagnosis of psychogenic pruritus

This section outlines a general diagnostic strategy for patients who:

- are complaining of a variable degree of pruritus;
- may or may not reveal the presence of excoriations on physical examination;
- have neither primary skin lesion nor any underlying organic disorder;
- have not had a neurological work-up.

(See Fig. 11.1.)

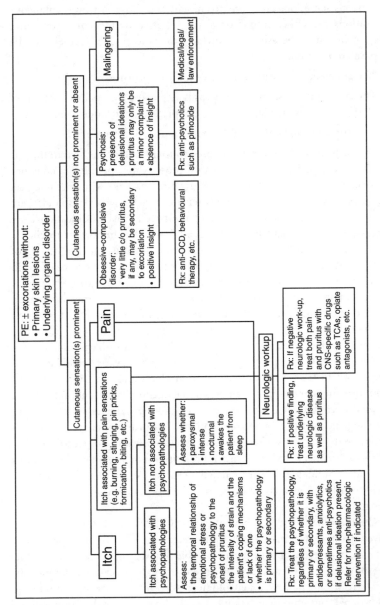

Fig. 11.1 Differential diagnosis of psychogenic pruritus.

Among this population, patients can be divided into those in whom cutaneous sensations are more prominent and those in whom cutaneous sensations are either minor or absent relative to the chief complaint (e.g. delusion of parasitosis, neurotic excoriation). The former may be separated into three categories.

- The cutaneous sensation consists entirely of pruritus.
- The cutaneous sensation of pruritus is associated with pain sensations of all types such as burning, stinging, pin pricks, formication, biting, etc.
- Pain turns out to be the predominant cutaneous sensation.

When pruritus presents as the predominant cutaneous sensation, it is useful to categorize these patients into those whose pruritus is or is not associated with psychopathology. Among those patients with psychological disturbances, the most commonly encountered psychopathologies are depression, anxiety, and a mixture of the two. Delusional ideation is an occasional concomitant finding.[2] In addition, it is important to elicit a temporal relationship between the onset of pruritus and the timing of emotional stress. It is even more important to evaluate the degree of strain in response to stress. As personalities and coping strategies vary greatly, the resultant strain in response to stressors in life also varies immensely from one person to another. Thus, knowledge of the intensity of strain on a patient and the coping mechanism in response to stress may be especially helpful in determining the need for adjunct, non-drug intervention. Finally, whether the psychopathologies are primary or secondary, it is important to treat them anyway with antidepressants, anxiolytic agents, and sometimes antipsychotics if delusional ideation is present (Table 11.1).

In this context, it is noteworthy that, among patients suffering from psychogenic pruritus, a major depressive disorder often presents with prominent symptoms of anxiety and agitation, leading often to misdiagnosis as a primary anxiety disorder. Prescription of anxiolytic medications instead of antidepressants can actually exacerbate the underlying depressive disorder,[19] as anxiolytics such as benzodiazepines generally have a depressant effect.[21]

On the other hand, for patients with pruritus but without associated psychopathology, it may be helpful to determine whether their pruritus is intense, paroxysmal, nocturnal, or capable of awaking the patient at night. In some cases, pruritus can be severe enough to cause insomnia. In this group of patients, neurological screening work-up should be considered and empirical treatment with doxepin or naltrexone may be considered. For the diagnosis and treatment of neuropathic pruritus see Chapter 10.

Obsessive–compulsive disorder

The other major 'branch' of the diagnostic strategy presented in Fig. 11.1 consists of those patients without cutaneous sensations as the most prominent clinical presentation. Cutaneous sensations such as pruritus may be secondary, may be entirely absent, and, when present, are much less prominent as a complaint relative to delusional ideation or obsessive–compulsive picking. Obsessive–compulsive disorder (OCD), psychosis, and malingering should be considered as the possible differential diagnoses.

Patients with OCD frequently present with excoriations and little or no complaint of pruritus (or pruritus only secondary to excoriations). A classic example is neurotic excoriation where the patient is driven to scratch, pick, or rub the skin compulsively in areas within the reach of hands. Although the activity does not make sense to the patient, he or she is usually fully aware of maladaptive activity but powerless to stop it. In general, patients with OCD typically have good insight into their own suffering. Classically, both obsession and compulsion should be observed, but obsessive ideation may be missing among patients with primary dermatological diseases. The main treatment involves medication such as clomipramine, fluoxetine, and fluvoxamine as well as behavioural therapy (Table 11.1). In contrast, psychotic patients are diagnosed by the presence of delusional ideation. Pruritus is often absent and, when present, constitutes only a very minor part of the complaint. Commonly encountered psychotic patients in the dermatological setting are not those with schizophrenia but rather those with monosymptomatic hypochondriacal psychosis (MHP), a common example of which is delusion of parasitosis. Antipsychotics such as pimozide are the treatment of choice. Finally, malingering patients who present with excoriations present a very difficult situation to manage, because malingering is officially not considered a psychiatric illness and the patient knows exactly what he or she wants to achieve from having a 'medical illness'. Needless to say, these patients would never voluntarily admit that they are malingering. If malingering were suspected, apart from supportive care to minimize secondary complications such as skin infection, the management involves more use of legal and law enforcement personnel as opposed to medical personnel.

Therapeutic options

The multitude of therapeutic options for pruritus suspected of having a psychogenic origin is divided into the following four categories.

- Behavioural and insight-oriented psychotherapy.
- CNS-specific pharmacological therapy (Table 11.1).

Table 11.1 Therapy of psychogenic pruritus

Aimed mechanism(s)	Drug	Starting dose/ schedule	Usual/maximal dose/ schedule	Adverse effects/precautions
Antidepressive with strongest H_1-receptor antagonism	Doxepin	25 mg t.d.s	Increase the dose by 25 mg after 1 week; maximal daily dose 300 mg	Sedation, cardiac conduction disturbances, weight gain, orthostatic hypotension, anticholinergic effect, lowered seizure threshold. Can be dangerous together with alcohol
Antidepressants with analgesic effects	Amitryptyline	25 mg o.d.	Increase the dose every 5–7 days. Usually one dose noctem will suffice	Sedation, dizziness, anticholinergic effect, tachycardia, lowered seizure threshold, sexual dysfunction. May not be appropriate choice in old and frail
Antidepressant with strong serotonin reuptake inhibition	Paroxetine	5–10 mg o.d.	20 mg o.d.	Nausea and vomiting, sedation, sexual dysfunction
Opioid antagonists, when opioidergic tone is increased	Naltrexone	25 mg o.d.	25–50 mg b.i.d.	Watch for opioid withdrawal syndrome: diarrhoea, nausea, vomiting, fatigue, and dizziness. This syndrome, which occurs initially, supports the idea of increased opioidergic tone. These symptoms usually disappear after one day.

Category	Drug	Dose	Titration	Adverse effects
Antipsychotics with analgesic	Pimozide	1–2 mg o.d.	Increase by 0.5–1 mg per week; maximal dose 6 mg o.d.; therapeutic dose to be maintained for at least 1 month; taper by 1 mg per week	Tardive dyskinesia, stiffness, restlessness (latter two may be treated with diphenhydramine 25 mg o.d.)
Anxiolytic and antidepressant	Alprazolam	0.125–0.5 mg t.d.s.	Increase by 0.125 mg per day; use for no more than 2–3 week; taper slowly	Sedation, addiction
Anxiolytic	Buspiron	5–10 mg t.d.s.	Maximal dose 50 mg/day	Non-addictive with long-term use. Adverse effects: nausea, diarrhoea, headache, restlessness, fatigue, and dizziness
Used in obsessive–compulsive disorder (OCD)	Clomipramine	25 mg o.d.	Increase weekly by 50 mg/day up to 300 mg/day	Lowered seizure threshold, sexual dysfunction, nausea, anticholinergic symptoms
	Fluoxetine	20 mg o.d.	Up to 60 mg o.d.	Diarrhoea, agitation, anxiety, and rash
	Fluvoxamine	25 mg b.i.d.	Up to 150 mg b.i.d.; increase by 50 mg/day increments	Nausea and vomiting

- Topical therapy is indicated only when pruritus and pain appear to be secondary to excoriations (see Chapter 12).
- Non-specific and supportive therapy (Box 11.1).

Specific information on the dosage and prominent side effects of CNS-specific pharmacotherapies is listed in Table 11.1.

Behavioural and insight-oriented psychotherapy

Welkowitz et al.[22] reported the first case of neurotic scratching successfully treated with a multicomponent behavioural programme consisting of self-monitoring, stimulus-control procedures and functional analyses all aimed at breaking scratching as a spinal reflex. To do so, such behavioural intervention attempts to break down a seemingly automatic behaviour (i.e. scratch) into its components and promote instructional procedures for controlling these elements, hence 'unlearning' the scratch response to stress (see Chapter 14). In addition to primary psychogenic pruritus, this behavioural approach may also be applicable to psychophysiological, pruritic dermatoses including lichen simplex chronicus[23] and atopic dermatitis.[24] In the case reported by Welkowitz et al.[22] treatment lasted 12 weeks, during which time scratching frequency markedly declined, and its gains were maintained up to a follow-up period of 6 months. This type of multicomponent behavioural programme has long been used successfully for Tourette's syndrome and, as compared to psychotherapy, is less time-consuming and perhaps more feasible for those patients resistant to exploring long-standing emotional issues. Yet, sometimes simply making

Box 11.1 Non-specific therapeutic options

- Cold compresses with moisturization
- Mentholated compounds, e.g. Sarna lotion
- Oral and topical antibiotics, if pruritus secondary to infection
- Occlusion, e.g. Unnaboot®, Duoderm®, boxing gloves
- Laser
- Cryotherapy
- Intralesional steroid injection
- Phototherapy (UVA, UVB, PUVA)
- Goeckerman therapy[22, 23]

the psychogenic pruritic patient aware of a possible causal relationship between emotional trauma and pruritus can 'cure' the patient. This has been illustrated by a rare form of psychogenic pruritus termed paroxysmal pruritus.[25, 26] As with psychogenic pruritus in general, paroxysmal pruritus can awaken the patient from sleep and, interestingly, can greatly elevate the threshold to the point that bleeding and ulceration would not be painful during acute episodes, predisposing to self-induced skin damage. However, for most patients falling into one of the diagnostic categories in Fig. 11.1, insight-oriented psychotherapy is usually much more involved.[3, 27–29] In an uncontrolled series of 63 cases of neurotic excoriation treated with psychotherapy, a low percentage success rate (13 of 63 patients) was reported.[3] Most other reports of psychotherapeutic success are case studies and thus anecdotal in nature.[27, 28]

Psychotropic drugs

Pharmacological therapies directed at psychopathologies such as depression, anxiety, OCD, and psychosis are discussed in depth elsewhere[21] and summarized in Table 11.1. Briefly, for psychogenic pruritus with underlying depression, the newer tricyclic antidepressant doxepin is recommended for both its antidepressive and antihistamine action profiles. In fact, doxepin is 775 times more potent as an H_1-antihistamine than diphenhydramine and 56 times more potent than hydroxyzine.[30] For psychogenic pruritus provoked by underlying anxiety, one can resort to either of two types of anti-anxiety medications: a quick-acting benzodiazepine that can potentially be sedating and a slow-acting non-benzodiazepine that is not dependency-producing or sedating. Among the former, the newer benzodiazepine alprazolam is recommended; among the latter, buspirone is the preferred choice. As opposed to most other benzodiazepines, alprazolam also has an antidepressant effect; this feature proves especially helpful since most psychodermatological patients have the agitating subtype of depression. Anti-OCD medications have been mentioned earlier and consist of antidepressants. For MHP, pimozide is the treatment of choice. Notably, pimozide also has an anti-opioid effect in addition to its anti-dopamine effect,[31] suggesting that it may also be helpful in treating pruritus secondary to self-induced trauma to the skin.

In practice, treatment of potential psychopathologies underlying psychogenic pruritus may not be successful, may be only partially successful, or may have a slow onset of efficacy. Hence, effective treatments aimed directly at the symptom of pruritus are often needed. In fact, most of the medications cited above for psychopathologies are recommended for their cross-acting efficacy directly against pruritus: doxepin for its potent antihistamine action, alprazolam for its sedating effect, and pimozide for its anti-opioid effect. Interestingly, sedation has been found to be critical in the antipruritic action of sedative H_1-antihistamines (e.g. diphenhydramine, tripelennamine, chlorphenamine, cyproheptadine, hydroxyzine). For instance, astemizole and terfenadine (low-sedative H_1-antihistamines) have been shown to have no effect on pruritus, whereas trimeprazine (sedating but less potent H_1-antihistamine) as well as nitrazepam (a sedating benzodiazepine) were shown to be antipruritic.[32] It was thus concluded that H_1-antihistamines have a peripheral antipruritic action in pruritoceptive type of pruritus (as in wealing disorders such as chronic idiopathic urticaria).[33, 34] In this context, it is noteworthy that doxepin (10 mg three times a day (ter die sumendus; t.d.s.)) has been shown to be much more effective in the treatment of chronic urticaria than diphenhydramine (25 mg t.d.s.).[35] Thus, although sedative H_1-antihistamines are effective in many patients with chronic urticaria (urticaria and pruritus lasting > 6 weeks), a sizeable minority of these patients does not obtain adequate relief of symptoms from these medications. It has been shown that as much as 70% of chronic urticaria is idiopathic and 16% is associated with severe depression or other psychiatric problems.[36]

As evident from our current understanding of the pathogenesis of pruritus in general and psychogenic pruritus in particular, while there are potentially many mediators and modulators of pruritus, the central mechanism(s) of pruritus remains largely unknown and a common final pathway elusive. CNS-specific therapeutic options are available, targeting some promising mechanisms. These options include opioid receptor antagonists (e.g. naloxone, nalmefene, and naltrexone) and selective serotonin 5-HT_3 receptor antagonists (e.g. ondansetron, tropisetron). Clinical and experimental observations have pointed to a role for centrally acting opioids in evoking or intensifying pruritus independently of their histamine-releasing effect.[37, 38] Naltrexone, an oral opioid receptor antagonist, was first shown to ameliorate intractable cholestatic pruritus and uraemic pruritus in double-blind and placebo-controlled trials (see Chapters 5 and 6).[39, 40] More recently, in open label pilot studies, naltrexone was shown to be highly antipruritic (i.e. improvement of 50% or more), with a total response rate of 70% within a week of administration, and well-tolerated in a variety of internal and dermatological diseases and among a patient population the majority of whom had failed other therapeutic options.[41, 42] In particular, naltrexone was found to be antipruritic in 9 out of 17 patients with prurigo nodularis. Among these 17 patients, 7 were diagnosed with psychogenic pruritus.[41]

Topical therapy

As mentioned earlier, doxepin exerts both central (i.e. antidepressant, sedative) and peripheral (i.e. H_1-antihistaminic) actions against pruritus (see Chapter 12). Thus, it is not surprising that the peripheral antipruritic action profile of doxepin has been capitalized on for the management of pruritic skin conditions. In experimentally induced (i.e. histamine-induced) pruritus, a 5% topical solution of doxepin was found to be more efficacious than topical amitriptyline, diphenhydramine, and the vehicle control.[43] In addition, doxepin cream 5% has been found to relieve pruritus in patients with atopic dermatitiis in a double-blind, vehicle-controlled, multicentre study.[44] As psychogenic pruritus represents a heterogeneous diagnostic group of patients, it is not clear at present whether topical doxepin has specific role in the management of patients with psychogenic pruritus.

EMLA (eutectic mixture of local anaesthetics) cream, has also been shown to be effective in increasing the threshold to experimentally induced pruritus, using histamine, cowhage, and papain, as compared to placebo.[45] It contains both lignocaine and prilocaine ointment. Other topical anaesthetics shown to be effective in experimental pruritus include pramoxine (1% lotion).[46] Topical pramoxine was shown to decrease both pruritus magnitude and duration while having no effect on thermal and pain thresholds. Furthermore, EMLA may have a role together with other topical agents in the management of pruritus. It has recently been shown that pre-treatment with EMLA significantly blocked the adverse effects of topical capsaicin (see below) such as burning and hyperalgia in experimental subjects.[47] It is unknown whether EMLA and capsaicin might have synergistic effects on pruritus, especially that of psychogenic or neurogenic origin.

Capsaicin, the pungent agent of red pepper, has been proposed to be effective in a wide variety of pruritic conditions by excitation of C-fibre afferents and the subsequent neuropeptide (such as SP) depletion, leading to skin desensitization to pruritic stimulation.[48] It has been shown to be efficacious for notalgia paraesthetica,[49, 50] brachioradial pruritus,[51, 52] and prurigo nodularis.[53] In the latter study, the causes of prurigo nodularis included psychogenic pruritus and generalized idiopathic pruritus in cases that were resistant to previous therapeutic attempts. Capsaicin cream 0.025% was administered twice daily (b.d.) under occlusion for the initial

3 days and subsequently raised in steps of 0.025% up to 0.3% every 3–5 days until total relief. Strikingly, complete remission of prurigo nodularis and pruritus was observed in all patients.[53] However, capsaicin use in clinical practice appears to be limited by its adverse effects such as burning and hyperalgesia.

Non-specific therapeutic options

Many non-specific treatment options exist to be used concomitantly with other more specific treatment agents aforementioned or, unfortunately in some cases, as measures of last resort (see Box 11.1). In all cases, one cannot ignore the fundamental importance of supportive care such as cold compresses with liberal moisturization. Such supportive care is soothing, provides hydration, facilitates debridement of crusts, and reduces xerosis, which may exacerbate pruritus. Mentholated compounds may also be helpful for symptomatic relief. When present, secondary bacterial infection must be treated aggressively with antibiotics. Moreover, occlusion can be helpful, given the cooperation of the patients. Pruritic lesions, such as those in prurigo nodularis resulting from chronic pruritus, may be removed by laser, cryotherapy, or even intralesional triamcinolone injection. Other measures that may play a role in the management of psychogenic pruritus include Goeckerman therapy[54, 55] and phototherapy with UVB or PUVA (psoralen plus ultraviolet A). The former therapy should be tried first.

Conclusions

- Up to 75% of dermatology patients have a significant psychogenic component to their skin complaints.
- Psychogenic pruritus is not a diagnosis of exclusion.
- Differential diagnosis of psychogenic pruritus should include neuropathic pruritus.
- Using the diagnosis of psychogenic pruritus for all pruritic conditions without primary skin changes is wrong and can be dangerous.
- Psychogenic pruritus is often paroxysmal and it frequently (but not always) ceases during sleep.
- Psychological depression and anxiety may amplify perception of any type of pruritus.
- Release of histamine and other vasoactive peptides from mast cells may be stimulated by psychological stress.

- Patients with obsessive–compulsive disorders frequently present with excoriations but only little or no pruritus.
- Therapy with psychotropic drugs reinforced by behavioural therapy is the mainstay of the therapy of psychogenic pruritus.
- Topical therapy is only of limited value in the treatment of psychogenic pruritus.

References

1. Weintraub E, Robinson C, Newmeyer M. (2000). Catastrophic medical complication in psychogenic excoriation. *South Med J* **93**:1099–101.
2. Koo JY, Do JH, Lee CS. (2000). Psychodermatology. *J Am Acad Dermatol* **43**:848–53.
3. Fruensgaard K. (1991). Psychotherapeutic strategy and neurotic excoriations. *Int J Dermatol* **30**:198–203.
4. Arnold LM, McElroy SL, Mutasim DF, Dwight MM, Lamerson CL, Morris EM. (1998). Characteristics of 34 adults with psychogenic excoriation. *J Clin Psychiatry* **59**:509–14.
5. Canavero S, Bonicalzi V, Massa-Micon B. (1997). Central neurogenic pruritus: a literature review. *Acta Neurol Belg* **97**:244–7.
6. Johnson RE, Kanigsberg ND, Jimenez CL. (2000). Localized pruritus: a presenting symptom of a spinal cord tumor in a child with features of neurofibromatosis. *J Am Acad Dermatol* **43**:958–61.
7. Gupta MA, Gupta AK, Kirkby S, *et al.* (1989). Pruritus associated with nocturnal wakenings: organic or psychogenic? *J Am Acad Dermatol* **21**:479–84.
8. Bernhard JD. (1990). Nocturnal wakening caused by pruritus: organic or psychogenic? *J Am Acad Dermatol* **23**:767.
9. Fried RG. (1994). Evaluation and treatment of 'psychogenic' pruritus and self-excoriation. *J Am Acad Dermatol* **30**:993–9.
10. Fjellner B, Arnetz BB. (1985). Psychological predictors of pruritus during mental stress. *Acta Derm Venereol* **65**:504–8.
11. Panconesi E, Hautmann G. (1996). Psychophysiology of stress in dermatology. The psychobiologic pattern of psychosomatics. *Dermatol Clin* **14**:399–421.
12. Gupta MA, Gupta AK. (1999). Depression modulates pruritus perception. A study of pruritus in psoriasis, atopic dermatitis and chronic idiopathic urticaria. *Ann NY Acad Sci* **885**:394–5.
13. Singh LK, Pang X, Alexacos N, Letourneau R, Theoharides TC. (1999). Acute immobilization stress triggers skin mast cell degranulation via corticotropin releasing hormone, neurotensin, and substance P: a link to neurogenic skin disorders. *Brain Behav Immun* **13**:225–39.

14. Koblenzer CS. (1992). Cutaneous manifestations of psychiatric disease that commonly present to the dermatologist—diagnosis and treatment. *Int J Psychiatry Med* **22**:47–63.

15. Cormia FE, Kuykendall V. (1953). Experimental histamine pruritus: nature, physical and environmental factors influencing development and sensitivity. *J Invest Dermatol* **20**:429–446.

16. Edwards AE, Shellow WV, Wright ET, Dignam TF. (1976). Pruritic skin diseases, psychological stress, and the itch sensation. A reliable method for the induction of experimental pruritus. *Arch Dermatol* **112**:339–43.

17. Gupta MA, Gupta AK, Kirkby S, *et al.* (1988). Pruritus in psoriasis. A prospective study of some psychiatric and dermatologic correlates. *Arch Dermatol* **124**:1052–7.

18. Gupta MA, Gupta AK, Schork NJ, Ellis CN. (1994). Depression modulates pruritus perception: a study of pruritus in psoriasis, atopic dermatitis, and chronic idiopathic urticaria. *Psychosom Med* **56**:36–40.

19. Gupta MA. (1995). Evaluation and treatment of 'psychogenic' pruritus and self-excoriation. *J Am Acad Dermatol* **32**:532–3.

20. Koblenzer CS. (1983). Psychosomatic concepts in dermatology. A dermatologist–psychoanalyst's viewpoint. *Arch Dermatol* **119**:501–12.

21. Koo JY, Pham CT. (1992). Psychodermatology. Practical guidelines on pharmacotherapy. *Arch Dermatol* **128**:381–8.

22. Welkowitz LA, Held JL, Held AL. (1989). Management of neurotic scratching with behavioral therapy. *J Am Acad Dermatol* **21**:802–4.

23. Roberston IM, Jordan JM, Whitlock FA. (1975). Emotions and skin (II)—the conditioning of scratch responses in cases of lichen simplex. *Br J Dermatol* **92**:407–12.

24. Gil KM, Sampson HA. (1989). Psychological and social factors of atopic dermatitis. *Allergy* **44** (Suppl. 9):84–9.

25. Arnold HL Jr. (1984). Paroxysmal pruritus. Its clinical characterization and a hypothesis of its pathogenesis. *J Am Acad Dermatol* **11**:322–6.

26. Hazelrigg DE. (1985). Paroxysmal pruritus. *J Am Acad Dermatol* **13**:839–40.

27. Koblenzer CS. (1986). Successful treatment of a chronic and disabling dermatosis by psychotherapy. A case report and discussion. *J Am Acad Dermatol* **15**:390–3.

28. Koblenzer CS. (1995). Psychotherapy for intractable inflammatory dermatoses. *J Am Acad Dermatol* **32**:609–12.

29. Koblenzer CS. (1996). Neurotic excoriations and dermatitis artefacta. *Dermatol Clin* **14**:447–55.

30. Richelson E. (1978). Tricyclic antidepressants block histamine H1 receptors of mouse neuroblastoma cells. *Nature* **274**:176–7.

31. Boublik JH, Funder JW. (1984). Interaction of dopamine receptor ligands with subtypes of the opiate receptor. *Eur J Pharmacol* **107**:11–16.

32. Krause L, Shuster S. (1983). Mechanism of action of antipruritic drugs. *Br Med J (Clin Res Ed)* **287**:1199–200.

33. Monroe EW, Bernstein DI, Fox RW, *et al.* (1992). Relative efficacy and safety of loratadine, hydroxyzine, and placebo in chronic idiopathic urticaria. *Arzneimittelforschung* **42**:1119–21.

34. Brostoff J, Fitzharris P, Dunmore C, Theron M, Blondin P. (1996). Efficacy of mizolastine, a new antihistamine, compared with placebo in the treatment of chronic idiopathic urticaria. *Allergy* **51**:320–5.

35. Greene SL, Reed CE, Schroeter AL. (1985). Double-blind crossover study comparing doxepin with diphenhydramine for the treatment of chronic urticaria. *J Am Acad Dermatol* **12**:669–75.

36. Juhlin L. (1981). Recurrent urticaria: clinical investigation of 330 patients. *Br J Dermatol* **104**:369–81.

37. Bernstein JE, Swift RM, Soltani K, Lorincz AL. (1982). Antipruritic effect of an opiate antagonist, naloxone hydrochloride. *J Invest Dermatol* **78**:82–3.

38. Fjellner B, Hägermark O. (1982). Potentiation of histamine-induced itch and flare responses in human skin by the enkephalin analogue FK-33–824, beta-endorphin and morphine. *Arch Dermatol Res* **274**:29–37.

39. Peer G, Kivity S, Agami O, *et al.* (1996). Randomised crossover trial of naltrexone in uraemic pruritus. *Lancet* **348**:1552–4.

40. Wolfhagen FH, Sternieri E, Hop WC, Vitale G, Bertolotti M, Van Buuren HR. (1997). Oral naltrexone treatment for cholestatic pruritus: a double-blind, placebo-controlled study. *Gastroenterology* **113**:1264–9.

41. Metze D, Reimann S, Luger TA. (1999). Effective treatment of pruritus with naltrexone, an orally active opiate antagonist. *Ann NY Acad Sci* **885**:430–2.

42. Metze D, Reimann S, Beissert S, Luger T. (1999). Efficacy and safety of naltrexone, an oral opiate receptor antagonist, in the treatment of pruritus in internal and dermatological diseases. *J Am Acad Dermatol* **41**:533–9.

43. Bernstein JE, Whitney DH, Soltani K. (1981). Inhibition of histamine-induced pruritus by topical tricyclic antidepressants. *J Am Acad Dermatol* **5**:582–5.

44. Drake LA, Fallon JD, Sober A. (1994). Relief of pruritus in patients with atopic dermatitis after treatment with topical doxepin cream. The Doxepin Study Group. *J Am Acad Dermatol* **31**:613–16.

45. Shuttleworth D, Hill S, Marks R, Connelly DM. (1988). Relief of experimentally induced pruritus with a novel eutectic mixture of local anaesthetic agents. *Br J Dermatol* **119**:535–40.

46. Yosipovitch G, Maibach HI. (1997). Effect of topical pramoxine on experimentally induced pruritus in humans. *J Am Acad Dermatol* **37**:278–80.

47. Yosipovitch G, Maibach HI, Rowbotham MC. (1999). Effect of EMLA pre-treatment on capsaicin-induced burning and hyperalgesia. *Acta Derm Venereol* **79**:118–21.

48. Lynn B. (1992). Capsaicin: actions on C fibre afferents that may be involved in itch. *Skin Pharmacol* 5:9–13.

49. Wallengren J. (1991). Treatment of notalgia paresthetica with topical capsaicin. *J Am Acad Dermatol* 24:286–8.

50. Wallengren J, Klinker M. (1995). Successful treatment of notalgia paresthetica with topical capsaicin: vehicle-controlled, double-blind, crossover study. *J Am Acad Dermatol* 32:287–9.

51. Knight TE, Hayashi T. (1994). Solar (brachioradial) pruritus—response to capsaicin cream. *Int J Dermatol* 33:206–9.

52. Goodless DR, Eaglstein WH. (1993). Brachioradial pruritus: treatment with topical capsaicin. *J Am Acad Dermatol* 29:783–4.

53. Stander S, Luger T, Metze D. (2001). Treatment of prurigo nodularis with topical capsaicin. *J Am Acad Dermatol* 44:471–8.

54. Armstrong RB, Leach EE, Fleiss JL, Harber LC. (1984). Modified Goeckerman therapy for psoriasis. A two-year follow-up of a combined hospital-ambulatory care program. *Arch Dermatol* 120:313–8.

55. Belsito DV, Kechijian P. (1982). The role of tar in Goeckerman therapy. *Arch Dermatol* 118:319–21.

12

Topical therapy

Jacek C. Szepietowski and Robert
Twycross

General principles

Topical agents are often the only therapy prescribed for many skin diseases. The total effect of the treatment with topical agents depends not only on the type and concentration of active substance, but also on the vehicle. The vehicle determines whether the topical therapy is drying or moisturizing and can also affect drug absorption. Thus, moist inflammatory lesions are treated with solutions, lotions, or gels to achieve a drying effect. However, using such vehicles is associated with low absorption of the active substance. In contrast, ointments are recommended for dry scaly lesions.[1, 2]

Several dermatoses are accompanied by pruritus (see Table 1.2). Pruritus is probably the most common symptom in dermatological patients.[3] It generally disappears spontaneously when the skin lesions improve.[4] However, topical agents that improve skin lesions, for example, corticosteroids, should not be regarded as antipruritic agents. In this chapter, attention is paid mainly to topical antipruritics that might help in the treatment of either localized or generalized pruritus. Some clinicians use only topical therapy for localized pruritus, whereas, if necessary for generalized pruritus, management may progress from topical to systemic therapy.[4]

It is essential to break the itch–scratch cycle to prevent secondary lichenification and so-called 'scratch lesions'. This can be achieved through a combination of non-drug and drug measures. Patients troubled by pruritus generally benefit from keeping their skin cold. Therefore, the following advice is recommended:

- wear light cool clothes;
- maintain a cool ambient environment that is not too dry (dryness of the skin should be avoided as it may provoke pruritus);
- have tepid showers or baths;
- avoid alcohol and hot or spicy foods and drinks.

Moreover, patients should be instructed to avoid contact with woollen products, and to keep their nails short (filed, not cut with scissors) to minimize damage of the skin due to scratching.[5, 6]

Emollients (moisturizers)

Dry skin (xerosis) is commonly associated with pruritus. The regular application of emollients is usually the first step in reducing the intensity of pruritus in many skin and systemic diseases.[6] Emollients should be applied to all pruritic areas of the skin at least twice daily. However, more frequent use, up to 4–6 times a day, is even more effective. Emollients should be put on the skin immediately after bathing.[4] Nowadays, many emollients are available. It is often sensible to recommend several products and allow the patient to choose the most comfortable one for them. The products should be dermatologically tested and contain no perfumes or other potential allergens.

Preparations containing urea 5–10% are frequently used. Urea is a naturally occurring moisturizing factor and helps to keep the stratum corneum of the epidermis adequately hydrated. Moreover, lipid preparations (e.g. ceramides) help because they restore epidermal lipids, thereby preventing increased transepidermal water loss.[7–9] A recent study confirmed significant relief of pruritus in patients with end-stage renal failure after the regular use of a hypo-irritant product containing 0.0005% nonanoic acid vanillylamide.[10] This resulted in a marked increase of the water content of epidermal stratum corneum. These observations support the role of emollients in the management of pruritus.

Special attention should also be paid to oil baths. Mineral and natural bath oil products are available. The bath should be lukewarm (water temperature about 37 °C), and the patients should avoid use of detergents. After 10–15 minutes the skin should be gently dried. Local anaesthetics such as polidocanol are sometimes added to oil products to intensify the antipruritic effect (see below). The effectiveness of oil baths containing polidocanol was first noted in patients with atopic dermatitis and with uraemic pruritus. Emollients can be applied in conjunction with any other topical or systemic treatments.

Other non-specific measures

There are several time-honoured topical antipruritic agents.[4-6] They include:

- menthol, 0.5–2%;
- phenol, 0.2–5%;
- camphor, 0.2–5%;
- coal tar, 3%-8%.

Frequently, they are available in lotions or creams containing other agents. They can also be added to aqueous creams and applied several times a day. For example, Castellani's paint (0.5% menthol and 5% salicylic acid in alcohol 70%) is used for pruritus mainly of intertriginous and anal regions.[4] Although menthol acts more as a topical anaesthetic than as a cooling agent,[11] it gives a sensation of cooling.[12] All the above substances may be used together with other cooling treatments, such as cold wet compresses, milk compresses, or aluminium salts. The formula of one of the extemporaneous, non-specific antipruritic lotions consists of:

- menthol, 0.5
- liquified phenol, 1.0
- zinc lotion to make it up to 100.

Crotamiton

Topical 10% crotamiton has a mild antiscabetic effect, and it is therefore sometimes regarded as an antipruritic agent. In a controlled trial no significant difference in the reduction of pruritus was found after the topical application of crotamiton and plain aqueous cream.[13] Crotamiton should not be regarded as a specific antipruritic drug.

Local anaesthetics

Modern local anaesthetics (cocaine analogues or derivatives) may be helpful in localized pruritus, such as notalgia paraesthetica or pruritus ani.[14] Their effect is usually faster in onset and more marked than that obtained with traditional topical anaesthetic compounds such as menthol or camphor.[12] Benzocaine and lidocaine are the most commonly used local anaesthetics. Apart from lidocaine these substances may be responsible for allergic contact dermatitis. However, recent data indicate that the allergic potency of local anaesthetics may be much lower than was previously thought.[13] Absorption is variable and, if large amounts are applied, they could cause a cardiac arrhythmia. Their use is best restricted to a few days. The antipruritic activity of a mixture of 2.5% lidocaine and 2.5% prilocaine (EMLA cream) has been clearly demonstrated.[14, 15] Moreover, creams or oil baths with polidocanol 3%, a non-ionic surfactant with local anaesthetic properties, reduce pruritus in atopic and uraemic patients.[16–18]

Specific topical antipruritics

Topical H_1-antihistamines

Topical H_1-antihistamines, such as diphenhydramine, promethazine, mepyramine, and dimetindene, are widely available. Among topical agents, dimetindene and especially doxepin have been established as effective antipruritic agents and have been found to relieve pruritus associated with atopic dermatitis and insect bites.[12, 19–24] Doxepin, marketed primarily as a tricyclic antidepressant, is a broad-spectrum H_1- and H_2-receptor antagonist. This may explain why it is helpful in circumstances in which classic H_1-antihistamines bring little relief. Doxepin 5% cream, should be applied three or four times daily to no more than 10% of the body surface. The maximal dose is 3 g per application. On average, the intensity of the pruritus is reduced by about half, sometimes with initial benefit apparent after 15 minutes and typically with increasing benefit during the first week. The possibility of allergic contact dermatitis limits the use of topical H_1-antihistamines.[23, 25–27]

Capsaicin

Capsaicin is a substance isolated from pepper plants of the genus *Capsicum*. Capsaicin has been demonstrated to relieve both pruritus and pain. Its main mechanism of action is depletion of neuropeptides, especially substance P, from cutaneous nerve endings. Moreover, capsaicin is known to cause atrophy of cutaneous C-fibres.[12, 28, 29] Capsaicin 0.025–0.075% cream is recommended mainly for localized pruritus, for example, notalgia paraesthetica.[30, 31] It is also effective in localized uraemic pruritus,[29] hydroxyethyl starch-induced pruritus,[32] and in pruritus associated with psoriasis.[33, 34] It should be applied 3–5 times a day to achieve maximum effect. Although capsaicin is apparently free from systemic toxicity, its local tolerance may be poor because patients, especially at the beginning of the treatment, frequently experience burning and stinging when it is applied.[12, 35] Because of this, capsaicin is used only for localized pruritus.

Miscellaneous

Strontium nitrate

Topical strontium nitrate 10–20% has potent antipruritic properties. Its application reduces the pruritus of facial peels.[36, 37] It probably works by selectively blocking neuronal transmission in C-fibres.[5]

Corticosteroids

Corticosteroid creams should not be regarded as topical antipruritic agents. They possess strong anti-inflammatory activity, and they are highly effective in the treatment of several non-infective pruritic dermatoses. The reduction of the intensity of pruritus is related to the improvement of skin lesions and is not due to a direct effect on pruritus sensation. Therefore, generally, the use of topical corticosteroids should be limited to itchy non-infective inflammatory dermatoses.[4, 6, 12] Some authors suggested that they could be helpful also in so-called 'itchy non-visible dermatoses', where there are no visible skin lesions but there is some histopathological evidence of inflammatory infiltrates in the upper dermis.[6]

Topical immunosuppressants

Two new topical immunosuppressive agents, tacrolimus and pimecrolimus, have recently been introduced. They both inhibit cytokines release from activated lymphocytes (mainly T cells) and mast cells. Tacrolimus additionally has a suppressive effect on the Langerhans cells.[38, 39] Tacrolimus and pimecrolimus are about 100 times more potent than cyclosporin. They are very effective in patients with atopic dermatitis. A reduction of pruritus is observed a few days after starting regular application, especially with pimecrolimus treatment.[38, 39] Moreover, topical tacrolimus significantly reduces uraemic pruritus.[40] Although the initial studies have showed promising results, randomized, controlled, double-blind trials are essential to evaluate the antipruritic activity of these new topical immunosuppressants.

Ultraviolet phototherapy

Ultraviolet B (UVB) phototherapy

Phototherapy, especially with UVB, is an effective therapy for different types of pruritus, for example, uraemic pruritus,[41–43] cholestatic pruritus,[44] and pruritus associated with AIDS.[45, 46] Although not proven, it is postulated that UVB therapy has an immunomodulatory effect on skin via one or more mechanisms:

• a direct effect on the synthesis of soluble mediators (as yet unidentified);

• modulation of the expression of cell-surface associated molecules;

• stimulation of cell apoptosis.[47]

UVB has been shown to reduce the number of cutaneous mast cells due to apoptosis and causes degeneration of cutaneous nerves.[48] UVB phototherapy is usually well tolerated. In pruritic uraemic patients, after a course lasting 30 days, the mean duration of remission is about 18 months. The treatment cycle may be repeated several times; patients usually respond quickly to repeat therapy.[43, 49]

Photochemotherapy

Photochemotherapy (psoralen + UVA), PUVA, is widely used in dermatology and was shown to be effective in several pruritic inflammatory dermatoses, for example, atopic dermatitis, lichen planus, psoriasis. Relief of pruritus related to polycythaemia vera,[50, 51] AIDS,[52] and aquagenic pruritus[53, 54] after PUVA therapy has also been reported.

Conclusions

• Emollients and other non-specific measures are always the first step in antipruritic therapy.

• 5% doxepin cream is an effective topical agent for localized pruritus.

• Capsaicin, administered to a limited area, can be effective in uraemic and several other types of pruritus.

• Topical immunosuppressants are new and promising agents in the treatment of skin diseases associated with pruritus.

• Ultraviolet B phototherapy is effective in the treatment of different types of pruritus.

References

1. Monti M, Motta S. (1999). Topical preparations and vehicles. In: Katsambas AD, Lotti TM. (eds.), *European handbook of dermatological treatments*, Berlin: Springer-Verlag, pp. 834–46.

2. Cislo M. (2002). Principles of topical therapy [in Polish]. In: Szepietowski J. (ed.), *Treatment of skin and sexually transmitted diseases*, Warszawa: PZWL, pp. 15–39.

3. Szepietowski J. (1999). Pruritus and its pathogenesis [in Polish]. *Dermatol Klin Zabieg* 1:45–8.

4. Ioannides D. (1999). Pruritus. In: Katsambas AD, Lotti TM. (eds.). *European handbook of dermatological treatments*, Berlin: Springer-Verlag, pp. 470–6.

5. Twycross R, Greaves MW, Handwerker H, *et al.* (2003). Itch: scratching more than the surface. *QJM* 96:7–26.

6. Szepietowski J, Reich A. (2002). Management of pruritus [in Polish]. *Dermatol Estetyczna* 4:251–6.

7. Imokawa G, Hattori M. (1985). A possible function of structural lipids in the water-holding properties of the stratum corneum. *J Invest Dermatol* 84:282–4.

8. Randazzo SD, Dinotta F. (1993). Dry skin: pathophysiology and treatment. *J Appl Cosmetol* 11:121–6.

9. Szepietowski J, Bialynicki-Birula R. (2002). Evaluation of the efficacy and tolerance of urea, ceramide and physiological lipids combination in the treatment of dry skin [in Polish]. *Dermatol Estetyczna* 4:171–7.

10. Suigiura M, Hayakawa R, Sugiura K, Ogawa H, Yamasaki C, Shamoto M. (2000). Clinical evaluation of hypo-irritant products containing 0.005% nonanoic acid vanillylamide (NVA) on the itching sensation of patients under dialysis. *Environ Dermatol* 7:110–20.

11. Bromm B, Scharein E, Darsow U, Ring J. (1995). Effects of menthol and cold on histamine-induced itch and skin reactions in man. *Neurosci Lett* 187:157–60.

12. Fleischer AB. (ed.). (2000). *The clinical management of itching*. New York: The Parthenon Publishing Group.

13. Smith EB, King CA, Baker MD. (1984). Crotamiton lotion in pruritus. *Int J Dermatol* 23:684–5.

14. Szepietowski J, Wasik G. (2002). Notalgia paresthetica a rare form of localized pruritus [in Polish]. *Przegl Dermatol* 89:215–17.

15. Shuttleworth D, Hill S, Marks R, Connelly DM. (1988). Relief of experimentally induced pruritus with a novel eutectic mixture of local anaesthetic agents. *Br J Dermatol* 119:535–40.

16. Vieluf D, Matthies C, Ring J. (1992). Dry and itchy skin therapy with a new preparation, containing urea and polidocanol [in German]. *Z Hautkrankh* 67:816–21.

17. Wasik F, Szepietowski J, Szepietowski T, Weyde W. (1996). Relief of uraemic pruritus after balneological therapy with a bath oil containing polidocanol (Balneum Hermal Plus). An open clinical study. *J Dermatol Treat* **7**:231–3.

18. Freitag G, Hoppner T. (1997). Results of a postmarketing drug monitoring survey with a polidocanol–urea preparation for dry, itching skin. *Curr Med Res Opin* **13**:529–37.

19. Geiger P. (1976). Topical treatment of pruritus with Fenistil-gel [in German]. *Schweiz Rundsch Med Prax* **65**:594–5.

20. Lever LR, Hill S, Dykes PJ, Marks R. (1991). Efficacy of topical dimetindene in experimentally induced pruritus and weal and flare reactions. *Skin Pharmacol* **4**:109–12.

21. Drake LA, Fallon JD, Sober A. (1994). Relief of pruritus in patients with atopic dermatitis after treatment with topical doxepin cream. The Doxepin Study Group. *J Am Acad Dermatol* **31**:613–16.

22. Drake LA, Millikan LE. (1995). The antipruritic effect of 5% doxepin cream in patients with eczematous dermatitis. Doxepin Study Group. *Arch Dermatol* **131**:1403–8.

23. Smith PF, Corelli RL. (1997). Doxepin in the management of pruritus associated with allergic cutaneous reactions. *Ann Pharmacother* **31**:633–5.

24. Greiding L, Moreno P. (1999). Doxepin incorporated into a dermatologic cream: an assessment of both doxepin antipruritic action and doxepin action as an inhibitor of papules, in allergen and histamine-caused pruritus. *Allergol Immunopathol (Madr)* **27**:265–70.

25. Valsecchi R, di Landro A, Pansera B, Cainelli T. (1994). Contact dermatitis from a gel containing dimethindene maleate. *Contact Dermatitis* **30**:248–9.

26. Bilbao I, Aguirre A, Vicente JM, Raton JA, Zabala R, Diaz Perez JL. (1996). Allergic contact dermatitis due to 5% doxepin cream. *Contact Dermatitis* **35**:254–5.

27. Taylor JS, Praditsuwan P, Handel D, Kuffner G. (1996). Allergic contact dermatitis from doxepin cream. One-year patch test clinic experience. *Arch Dermatol* **132**:515–18.

28. Lynn B. (1992). Capsaicin: actions on C fibre afferents that may be involved in itch. *Skin Pharmacol* **5**:9–13.

29. Breneman DL, Cardone JS, Blumsack RF, Lather RM, Searle EA, Pollack VE. (1992). Topical capsaicin for treatment of hemodialysis-related pruritus. *J Am Acad Dermatol* **26**:91–4.

30. Wallengren J. (1991). Treatment of notalgia paresthetica with topical capsaicin. *J Am Acad Dermatol* **24**:286–8.

31. Leibsohn E. (1992). Treatment of notalgia paresthetica with capsaicin. *Cutis* **49**:335–6.

32. Szeimies RM, Stolz W, Wlotzke U, Korting HC, Landthaler M. (1994). Successful treatment of hydroxyethyl starch-induced pruritus with topical capsaicin. *Br J Dermatol* **131**:380–2.

33. Arnold WP, van de Kerkhof PC. (1994). Topical capsaicin in pruritic psoriasis. *J Am Acad Dermatol* **31**:135.

34. Ellis CN, Berberian B, Sulica VI, Dodd WA, Jarratt MT, Katz HI, Prawer S, Krueger G, Rex IH Jr, Wolf JE. (1993). A double-blind evaluation of topical capsaicin in pruritic psoriasis. *J Am Acad Dermatol* **29**:438–42.

35. Szepietowski J. (2002). Pruritus [in Polish]. In: Szepietowski J. (ed.), *Treatment of skin and sexually transmitted diseases*, Warszawa: PZWL, pp. 182–8.

36. Zhai H, Hannon W, Hahn GS, Pelosi A, Harper RA, Maibach HI. (2000). Strontium nitrate suppresses chemically-induced sensory irritation in humans. *Contact Dermatitis* **42**:98–100.

37. Zhai H, Hannon W, Hahn GS, Harper RA, Pelosi A, Maibach HI. (2000). Strontium nitrate decreased histamine-induced itch magnitude and duration in man. *Dermatology* **200**:244–6.

38. Cheer SM, Plosker GL. (2001). Tacrolimus ointment. A review of its therapeutic potential as a topical therapy in atopic dermatitis. *Am J Clin Dermatol* **2**:389–406.

39. Wellington K, Jarvis B. (2002). Topical pimecrolimus: a review of its clinical potential in the management of atopic dermatitis. *Drugs* **62**:817–40.

40. Pauli-Magnus C, Klumpp S, Alscher DM, Kuhlmann U, Mettang T. (2000). Short-term efficacy of tacrolimus ointment in severe uremic pruritus. *Perit Dial Int* **20**:802–3.

41. Gilchrest BA, Rowe JW, Brown RS, Steinman TI, Arndt KA. (1977). Relief of uremic pruritus with ultraviolet phototherapy. *N Engl J Med* **297**:136–8.

42. Imazu LE, Tachibana T, Danno K, Tanaka M, Imamura S. (1993). Histamine-releasing factor(s) in sera of uraemic pruritus patients in a possible mechanism of UVB therapy. *Arch Dermatol Res* **285**:423–7.

43. Urbonas A, Schwartz RA, Szepietowski JC. (2001). Uremic pruritus—an update. *Am J Nephrol* **21**:343–50.

44. Rosenthal E, Diamond E, Benderly A, Etzioni A. (1994). Cholestatic pruritus: effect of phototherapy on pruritus and excretion of bile acids in urine. *Acta Paediatr* **83**:888–91.

45. Lim HW, Vallurupalli S, Meola T, Soter NA. (1997). UVB phototherapy is an effective treatment for pruritus in patients infected with HIV. *J Am Acad Dermatol* **37**:414–17.

46. Schoppelrey HP, Breit R. (1999). UV-therapy in HIV-infected patients [in German]. *Hautarzt* **50**:643–8.

47. Krutmann J, Morita A. (1999). Mechanisms of ultraviolet (UV) B and UVA phototherapy. *J Investig Dermatol Symp Proc* **4**:70–2.

48. Szepietowski JC, Morita A, Tsuji T. (2002). Ultraviolet B induces mast cell apoptosis: a hypothetical mechanism of ultraviolet B treatment for uraemic pruritus. *Med Hypotheses* **58**:167–70.

49. Szepietowski JC, Schwartz RA. (1998). Uremic pruritus. *Int J Dermatol* **37**:247–53.

50. Swerlick RA. (1985). Photochemotherapy treatment of pruritus associated with polycythemia vera. *J Am Acad Dermatol* **13**:675–7.

51. Jeanmougin M, Rain JD, Najean Y. (1996). Efficacy of photochemotherapy on severe pruritus in polycythemia vera. *Ann Hematol* **73**:91–3.

52. Gorin I, Lessana-Leibowitch M, Fortier P, Leibowitch J, Escande JP. (1989). Successful treatment of the pruritus of human immunodeficiency virus infection and acquired immunodeficiency syndrome with psoralens plus ultraviolet A therapy. *J Am Acad Dermatol* **20**:511–13.

53. Smith RA, Ross JS, Staughton RC. (1994). Bath PUVA as a treatment for aquagenic pruritus. *Br J Dermatol* **131**:584.

54. Holme SA, Anstey AV. (2001). Aquagenic pruritus responding to intermittent photochemotherapy. *Clin Exp Dermatol* **26**:40–1.

13

Systemic therapy: making rational choices

Robert Twycross and Zbigniew Zylicz

The scope of this chapter

This chapter provides an overview of systemic therapy for pruritus. It assumes that, when indicated:

- topical measures are being used, for example, the regular application by patients with dry skin of an emollient (moisturizer) twice daily or more;

- correctable causes or exacerbating factors are being treated with appropriate disease-specific therapy, for example, stenting of the common bile duct in patients with obstructive cholestasis caused by cancer of the head of the pancreas;

- lifestyle changes have been introduced (Box 13.1).

The chapter consists of two parts concerning: drugs with antipruritic properties; cause-specific therapy.

Drugs with antipruritic properties

Histaminergic drugs

H_1-receptor antagonists

These drugs are also referred to as H_1-antihistamines. They are the drugs of choice for histamine-mediated pruritus. Chlorphenamine (sedative) 4 mg t.d.s. or cetirizine (low-sedative) 5 mg b.d. or 10 mg o.d. are commonly used. After relief is obtained, a lower maintenance dose may suffice.

Box 13.1 Keep cool! Healthy hints for people with pruritus

1. Avoid excessive heat (and cutaneous vasodilatation):
   - maintain a cool ambient environment that is not too dry;
   - wear light-weight clothes, preferably cotton;
   - have tepid showers or baths;
   - avoid alcohol and spicy food/drinks.
2. Ask each patient about possible idiosyncratic exacerbating factors; learn how to avoid them.
3. Reduce the likelihood of scratching and excoriation:
   - keep finger nails short, preferably by filing, not by cutting;
   - if desperate, rub pruritic areas gently with fingers; don't scratch with finger nails;
   - apply bland ointment to decrease skin damage by scratching and rubbing.

Any benefit in pruritus *not* mediated by histamine is associated with the sedative effect of the first-generation H_1-antihistamines; second- and third-generation low-sedative drugs have no effect.[1] In some studies, benzodiazepines were as beneficial as sedative H_1-antihistamines.[2] However, in one study, diazepam was no better than placebo.[3] In a study of pruritus associated with various dermatoses, amylobarbital was as effective as trimeprazine, an H_1-antihistamine.[4] However, another study demonstrated no benefit with barbiturates.[2]

H_2-receptor antagonists

Cimetidine, an H_2-receptor antagonist, enhances the effect of H_1-antihistamines in urticaria.[5, 6] In Hodgkin's lymphoma, case reports suggest that cimetidine, an H_2-receptor antagonist, 1 g daily in divided dosage, may be beneficial.[7] It may also be of benefit in polycythaemia vera.[8] The antipruritic effect may be related to inhibition of hepatic cytochrome CYP2D6, and will not be seen with ranitidine or famotidine.[9]

Mixed H_1- and H_2-receptor antagonist: doxepin

Doxepin, marketed primarily as a tricyclic antidepressant, is a potent H_1- and H_2-receptor antagonist. Its affinity for H_2 receptors is six times that of cimetidine.[10] It also blocks muscarinic receptors.[11] Amitriptyline is similar in potency to doxepin as an H_1-antihistamine, but other tricyclic antidepressants are much less so.[12] Patients with chronic urticaria who do not respond to conventional H_1-antihistamines may well benefit from doxepin 10–75 mg o.n.[11]

Doxepin is also available as a 5% cream.[13] It is of benefit in some patients with atopic dermatitis[14–16] but is not generally suitable for use in children (see Chapter 12). It is applied t.d.s. or q.d.s. to no more than 10% of the body surface. The maximum topical dose is 3 g per application. Absorption is variable and plasma concentrations range from undetectable to the same as the peak concentrations seen after doxepin 75 mg by mouth. So it is not clear whether the benefit can be ascribed to the topical or the systemic effect of the drug. On average, the intensity of the pruritus is reduced by about half, sometimes with initial benefit apparent after 15 minutes and typically with increasing benefit during the first week. About 15% of patients complain initially of localized stinging or burning, and a similar number of drowsiness. These symptoms generally decrease in time. Dry mouth can be a problem. Doxepin cream is not as effective as systemic treatment.[17] It is also expensive compared with doxepin tablets plus aqueous cream.

As with all tricyclic antidepressants, monoamine oxidase inhibitors should be discontinued at least 2 weeks before starting treatment with either topical or systemic doxepin. Patients prescribed doxepin by either route should also avoid the concurrent use of drugs that inhibit cytochrome P450, for example, cimetidine, imidazoles, antifungals, and macrolide antibiotics.

Serotoninergic drugs

5-HT_3 receptor antagonists
In patients with pruritus induced by spinal opioids, a randomized placebo-controlled trial of intravenous (IV) ondansetron 8 mg demonstrated benefit in 70% of patients within 1 hour.[18] Excellent results have also been reported in case reports and from open-label studies of either single or multiple doses of IV and/or oral ondansetron in chronic cholestasis and uraemia.[19–22] However, in randomized controlled trials, ondansetron was either of no[23] or minimal benefit[24] in cholestasis and uraemia.[25] In some centres, tropisetron 1–2 mg subcutaneously (SC) is used p.r.n. in dying patients with pruritus of cholestasis who cannot swallow.

Paroxetine

Paroxetine, a selective serotonin reuptake inhibitor (SSRI), relieves pruritus in some patients. Originally, a beneficial effect was noted in a patient with lung cancer and bullous pemphigoid who was given paroxetine for depression precipitated by intense pruritus.[26] Similar benefit was seen in two patients in whom the cause of the pruritus was paraneoplastic (cancers of the colon and prostate) and in two patients with morphine-induced pruritus. In a subsequent randomized controlled trial mainly in cancer patients, using a numerical scale (0–10), 37% of the patients reported at least 50% improvement with paroxetine 20 mg o.d. (Zylicz Z, Krajnik M, van Sorge AA, Costantini M. (2003). Paroxetine in the treatment of severe non-dermatological pruritus: a randomized, controlled trial. *J Pain Symptom Manage* (in press)). Relief usually occurred within 3 days, that is, too soon for the benefit to be secondary to the relief of depression. Of the responders, half to two-thirds experienced sedation or nausea; the latter responding to low doses of cisapride, that is, 5 mg b.d. Non-responders had significantly fewer adverse effects. Doses of paroxetine as low as 5–10 mg o.d. are now being used; such doses appear to be equally effective and reduce undesirable effects. Nausea and vomiting are successfully treated with 5-HT$_3$ antagonists. The benefit of paroxetine has been confirmed by a second group of investigators.[27, 28] In their experience no tolerance has been observed (Tefferi A, personal communication).

Because benefit has not yet been observed with other SSRIs, it is possible that paroxetine exerts its effect by a non-serotoninergic mechanism.

Mirtazapine

Mirtazapine, a noradrenaline and specific serotonin antidepressant with H$_1$-antihistamine properties,[29, 30] has been used successfully to relieve pruritus in patients with malignant cholestasis, lymphoma, and uraemia.[31] Doses of 15–30 mg o.n. were used but success with a dose of 7.5 mg has been reported (Zylicz Z, personal communication). It is possible that the antipruritic effect of mirtazapine is at least partly a consequence of non-specific sedation. On the other hand, it is both a 5-HT$_2$- and a 5-HT$_3$-receptor antagonist (as well as an H$_1$-antihistamine) and its antipruritic effect could be mediated wholly via serotoninergic mechanisms. Because of the anti-serotoninergic effects, the use of mirtazapine is not associated with initial nausea and vomiting.

Opioid antagonists

The use of opioid antagonists is discussed individually in the sections on cholestasis (see Chapter 5), uraemia (see Chapter 6), and the spinal administration of opioids (see Chapter 7). However, in an open-label uncontrolled study in various dermatological and systemic disorders, a good result was obtained in about 70% of the patients.[32] The results should be interpreted with caution in the absence of controlled data.

Cause-specific therapy

The next section is summarized in Table 13.1. However, because of a paucity of controlled studies with antipruritics, 'weight of evidence' is not the only criterion that determines a treatment of choice. Absence of hard evidence, for example, from a controlled trial, is not proof of lack of efficacy.

Cholestasis

Opioid antagonists

In controlled studies, both naloxone infusions[33–35] and oral nalmefene[30, 36, 37] have been shown to decrease scratching activity by patients with pruritus associated with cholestasis. Naloxone infusions have a potential place in the emergency treatment of acute exacerbations of the pruritus of cholestasis.[33, 34, 38] Naltrexone and nalmefene, which are both bioavailable by mouth, can be used subsequently.[30, 36, 37, 39–41] However, orally administered opioid antagonists can precipitate a transient opioid withdrawal-like reaction in patients with cholestasis including hallucinations and dysphoria.[42–45] To avoid or minimize such a reaction, treatment is best started with a cautious infusion of naloxone, for example, 0.002 µg/kg/min (about 160–200 µg/24 h).[44] The rate of infusion can be doubled every 3–4 h provided no withdrawal-like symptoms occur. After 18–24 h, when a rate known to be associated with opioid antagonistic effects is reached (0.2 µg/kg/min), the infusion is stopped and naltrexone 12.5 mg (one-quarter of a 50 mg tablet) t.d.s. or 25 mg (one-half of a 50 mg tablet) b.d. is started.[43, 44] The dose is escalated steadily over a few days until a satisfactory clinical response is obtained. At this stage the effective dose should be consolidated into a single daily maintenance dose. The dose range for naltrexone is 25–250 mg o.d.[44] Naltrexone is sometimes associated with hepatotoxicity.[46] The dose range for nalmefene is 25–120 mg o.d.[36] However, this drug is not available in Europe.

Opioid partial agonists

Buprenorphine, a partial µ-opioid receptor agonist and κ-opioid receptor antagonist and a weak δ-opioid receptor agonist, has been reported

Table 13.1 Management of itch in non-skin diseases and weight of evidence[a]

Condition	Step 1	Step 2	Step 3
General measures[b]	*Correct the correctable*, e.g. treat skin disorders	Emollient cream o.d.–b.d.	Sedative, e.g. benzodiazepine or sedative H_1-antihistamine e.g. chlorphenamine 4 mg t.d.s.
Uraemia[c]	UVB phototherapy (A) or (if localized) capsaicin cream 0.025–0.075% o.d.–b.d. (A)	Naltrexone 50 mg o.d. (A)[d]	Thalidomide 100 mg o.n. (A)[e]
Cholestasis[f]	Naltrexone 12.5–250 mg o.d. (A)	Rifampicin 75–300 mg o.d. (A) or paroxetine 5–20 mg o.d. (A)	Methyltestosterone 25 mg SL o.d. (C) or alternative, e.g. danazol 200 mg o.d.–t.d.s. (U)[g]
Hodgkin's lymphoma[h]	Prednisolone 10–20 mg t.d.s.	Cimetidine 800 mg/24 h (B)	Mirtazapine 15–30 mg o.n. (U)
Polycythaemia vera[h]	Aspirin 100–300 mg o.d. (A)	Paroxetine 5–20 mg o.d. (A)	Sedative, e.g. benzodiazepine
Spinal opioid-induced pruritus	Bupivacaine intrathecal (A)	NSAID: diclofenac 100 mg PR (A) or tenoxicam 20 mg IV (A)	Ondansetron 8 mg IV stat (A)
Paraneoplastic pruritus[h]	Paroxetine 5–20 mg o.d. (A)	Mirtazapine 15–30 mg o.n. (U)	Thalidomide 100 mg o.n. (U)[e]
Other causes or origin unknown	Paroxetine 5–20 mg o.d. (A)	Mirtazapine 15–30 mg o.n. (U)	Thalidomide 100 mg o.n. (U)[e]

a Weight of evidence based on the system used by the Agency for Healthcare Policy and Research, USA: (A) at least one randomized controlled trial; (B) non-randomized studies; (C) based on expert opinion and consensus reports; (U) unclassified, based on single case reports or small series.

b Non-specific measures can be taken independently of specific treatment.

c After the haemodialysis regimen has been optimized.

d Controlled trials give contradictory results (much benefit versus no benefit).

e Thalidomide is unlicensed and may cause severe neuropathy if used long-term.

f In total bile obstruction, where bile duct stenting is impossible or unwanted.

g Androgens may be hepatotoxic and may increase cholestasis while reducing pruritus.

h Assuming that cytoreductive/anticancer treatment is impossible or unwanted.

beneficial in two out of five patients with pruritus associated with cholestasis.[47] These observations suggest that there could be a specific range of increased opioidergic tone associated with pruritus. The use of a partial μ-opioid receptor antagonist may be advantageous, because withdrawal-like symptoms will not be precipitated. Similar effects can be sometimes observed with weak opioids. One patient with pruritus associated with primary biliary cirrhosis obtained relief from regular oral codeine.[48] Pruritus returned when codeine was stopped because of constipation. It was restarted with appropriate laxatives, and the patient has now had good relief from pruritus for over 3 years (Jones EA, personal communication).

Hepatic enzyme inducers

Rifampicin is widely used for pruritus associated with intrahepatic cholestasis.[49] It is a known inducer of mixed function oxidases and inhibitor of bile-acid reuptake from the gut[50, 51] and was used in a placebo-controlled trial in nine patients suffering from pruritus of cholestasis for 2 weeks. All patients reported significant reduction of pruritus after 1 week of treatment. The dose used ranged from 300 to 450 mg per day. By interrupting the enterohepatic circulation of bile acids, rifampicin may reduce the impact of increased bile acids on the metabolic processes of the liver. Rifampicin causes hepatic dysfunction in some patients, but the risk of this is reduced by starting with a low dose, for example, 75 mg o.d. If this is not effective after a week, the dose should be increased to 150 mg o.d., and then to 150 mg b.d.

Phenobarbital, another hepatic enzyme inducer, is also of benefit in a dose of 2–5 mg/kg/24 h.[52] However, any benefit is probably the result of non-specific sedation, and it is now seldom used.

Colestyramine

Colestyramine is an intestinally active anion exchange resin primarily licensed for the management of hypercholesterolaemia. However, by chelating bile acids in the intestines, it interrupts the enterohepatic circulation of bile acids. It has been used for many years to relieve pruritus in cholestatic disorders such as primary biliary cirrhosis.[53] Benefit has been claimed only in an open-label non-randomized long-term study of 27 patients.[54] Colestyramine is not effective in pruritus associated with complete large duct biliary obstruction because bile acids (and possibly other biliary pruritogens) do not reach the gut.

When used, one 4 g sachet is given before and one after breakfast so that the arrival of the resin in the duodenum coincides with gall bladder contraction.[54] If necessary, further doses can be taken before the midday and evening meals. The maintenance dose is generally 12 g per day. However, many patients find it unpalatable and nauseating, and it commonly causes bloating and constipation. For these reasons it is seldom used in terminal cancer patients. If used long-term, it can cause malabsorption of the fat-soluble vitamins A, D, E, and K.

Androgens

The use of androgens to relieve pruritus in cholestasis stems from the serendipitous observation some 60 years ago in a patient with primary biliary cirrhosis whose pruritus cleared up when given an androgen for an unrelated reason.[55] Benefit is largely limited to 17α-alkyl androgens, for example, norethandrolone, methyltestosterone, and stanozolol,[56] possibly because of their greater bioavailability.

Typical doses are:

- methyltestosterone 25 mg SL o.d.;
- norethandrolone 10 mg b.d.–t.d.s.;
- stanozolol 5–10 mg o.d.

The manufacture in the UK of the first two drugs was discontinued many years ago, and stanozolol was withdrawn worldwide in 2002. However, the antipruritic effect appears to be a class property, and benefit should be obtained with an alternative 17α-alkyl androgen, for example, danazol, fluoxymesterone, or oxandrolone. In women with a normal or long life expectancy, masculinization (amenorrhoea, hirsutism, and deepening of the voice) is a problem, but can be contained by reducing the dose of the androgen from daily to thrice weekly or even less.[56]

17α-alkyl androgens are directly toxic to hepatocytes.[57] It is possible that the effect of androgens like methyltestosterone and stanozolol is mediated via focal hepatocellular damage, thereby limiting the ability of the cholestatic liver to produce enkephalins.[58] Certainly, androgens themselves can cause cholestatic jaundice and have occasionally caused serious liver impairment.[59] This is clearly a potential problem for patients with a prognosis measured in years, for example, those with primary biliary cirrhosis.

Now that orally administered opioid antagonists are available, the use of androgens has been largely superseded, except perhaps in patients taking opioid analgesics for pain relief in advanced cancer (see Chapter 5). In such patients, a trial of a 17α-alkyl androgen for 7–10 days is warranted.

Uraemia

Enhancing the dialysis regimen is the standard response when dialysis patients experience pruritus. Parathyroidectomy may result in a remission of pruritus in patients with secondary hyperparathyroidism and hyper-calcaemia.[60] In other circumstances hypercalcaemia is not associated with pruritus.

Ultraviolet B phototherapy

Ultraviolet B therapy, particularly narrow-band UVB, is effective in many patients[61] and may be superior to drug therapy (see Chapter 12).[61, 62]

Opioid antagonists

The results with naltrexone are confusing. Both reported trials were randomized placebo-controlled double-blind studies of naltrexone 50 mg once daily, and both used visual analogue scales (VAS) as a subjective mea-sure of pruritus.[63, 64] Both studies involved small number of patients (15 and 23, respectively), and the results were consistently distinct. In the positive outcome trial, the patients had initial VAS scores of 90–100 mm, whereas in the negative outcome trial the mean initial VAS score was about 60 mm before the first 4 week period and about 50 mm before the second period. It is possible, therefore, that naltrexone is of benefit only in very severe uraemic pruritus, when a disturbance in the balance of μ-and κ-opioid receptors could become a prominent causal or exacerbating factor. Thus, until further data are available, it seems reasonable to offer a trial of naltrexone to uraemic patients with severe uncontrolled pruritus, possibly increasing the dose progressively to 250 mg/day (as in cholestasis) if 50 mg/day does not suffice.

Thalidomide

Thalidomide is effective in over 50% of patients.[65] However, because of its poor availability and potential for neuropathy, thalidomide should not be used unless other measures fail.

Haematological diseases

The use of α-interferon as a cytoreductive agent in polycythaemia vera is associated with amelioration of pruritus.[66, 67] Pruritus in polycythaemia vera responds poorly to H_1-antihistamines but often responds well to paroxetine.[28] However, the drug of choice is low-dose aspirin; 300 mg is generally effective within 30 minutes with a duration of action of 12–24 hours.[68–70] Because platelet degranulation is increased in polycythaemia vera (releasing serotonin and prostanoids) and is known to be decreased by aspirin, the antipruritic effect of aspirin could be related to its impact on platelet dynamics.[68]

Curative radiotherapy and/or chemotherapy is obviously the best approach in Hodgkin's lymphoma. Corticosteroids often relieve pruritus in late-stage Hodgkin's lymphoma, although the mechanism of this effect is unknown. In the past some patients obtained benefit with α-interferon,[71] but this treatment is no longer used. Paroxetine appears to be ineffective in Hodgkin's lymphoma (Zylicz Z, personal communication).

Solid tumours

Paraneoplastic pruritus associated with solid tumours is not eased by corticosteriods or cimetidine. However, paroxetine is almost always beneficial, often within 24 hours.[26]

HIV/AIDS

There are many causes of pruritus in HIV+ patients.[72] Treatment depends on the cause but, when not associated with skin disease or infestation, it is largely empirical. Some patients obtain benefit from indometacin 25 mg t.d.s.[73]

Opioid-induced pruritus

H_1-antihistamines are ineffective for opioid-induced pruritus caused by spinal opioids (see Chapter 7). Bupivacaine added to spinal opioids tends to restrict pruritus to just the face.[74] 5-HT_3-receptor antagonists, for example, ondansetron 4–8 mg IV, may also be beneficial.[18] In 100 patients treated in a controlled trial, relief was rapid and complete; usually within minutes. However, it is unclear if this effect is maintained later and if oral medication is equally beneficial.

Naloxone abolishes pruritus induced by spinal morphine but sometimes also reverses analgesia.[75–77] Pruritus associated with systemic morphine is similarly abolished. Naltrexone is also effective.[78] However, nalbuphine, a mixed μ-opioid receptor antagonist and κ-opioid receptor agonist, is more effective than naloxone and does not reverse analgesia.[79]

Intranasal and epidural butorphanol reduces spinal opioid-induced pruritus,[80–82] although when given alone it can induce pruritus.[83] Butorphanol, a potent $μ_1$- and $κ_1$-opioid receptor agonist and a weak $μ_2$-receptor agonist, may act as a competitive antagonist at μ_2-receptors when given with other opioids.

In one trial, IV propofol relieved pruritus induced by spinal morphine in over 80% of patients (compared to 16% in the placebo group),[84] but other studies have produced negative results.[78]

Pretreatment with a nonsteroidal anti-inflammatory drug (NSAID), either diclofenac 100 mg PR (per rectum) or IV tenoxicam 20 mg, has been shown to reduce the incidence, intensity, and duration of pruritus in surgical patients receiving spinal opioids.[85, 86] These patients also had significantly less pain than control patients and needed significantly less postoperative opioid analgesia. It is possible that the difference in opioid dosage may explain the difference between the two groups.

Opioid-induced pruritus is rare in palliative care; because few patients receive spinal opioids and those who do are not opioid-naïve. Further, such patients almost always receive bupivacaine concurrently. When pruritus is induced by a systemic opioid, switching to an alternative may help, for example, morphine to hydromorphone.[81, 82, 87]

Conclusions

- Intractable pruritus deserves the same degree of attention as pain.
- The pathogenesis of pruritus varies, ranging from a lack of moisture in the skin to a complex array of factors in uraemia.
- Treatment should be aimed at:
  - decreasing the peripheral irritation of pruritus receptors, for example, emollients, H_1-antihistamines (when indicated), and NSAIDs;
  - decreasing the transmission of pruritic impulses. This can be achieved by discontinuing exogenous pruritogens (e.g. opioids);
  - modifying the disease process (e.g. modify dialysis regimen);
  - antagonism (e.g. naltrexone);
  - depressing transmission (e.g. bupivacaine or doxepin).
- When such options are ineffective, paroxetine and probably mirtazapine should be considered.
- Alternatively, a sedative drug could be tried, whether a benzodiazepine or a sedative H_1-antihistamine.
- In relation to uraemic pruritus in particular, UVB phototherapy must not be forgotten.

References

1. Krause L, Shuster S. (1983). Mechanism of action of antipruritic drugs. *Br Med J* (*Clin Res Ed*) **287**:1199–200.

2. Muston H, Felix R, Shuster S. (1979). Differential effect of hypnotics and anxiolytics on itch and scratch. *J Invest Dermatol* **72**:283.

3. Hägermark O. (1973). Influence of antihistamines, sedatives, and aspirin on experimental itch. *Acta Derm Venereol* **53**:363–8.

4. Hellier F. (1963). A comparative trial of trimeprazine and amylobarbitone in pruritus. *Lancet* **1**:471–2.

5. Monroe EW, Cohen SH, Kalbfleisch J, Schulz CI. (1981). Combined H1 and H2 antihistamine therapy in chronic urticaria. *Arch Dermatol* **117**:404–7.

6. Bleehen SS, Thomas SE, Greaves MW, Newton J, Kennedy CT, Hindley F, Marks R, Hazell M, Rowell NR, Fairiss GM, *et al.* (1987). Cimetidine and chlorpheniramine in the treatment of chronic idiopathic urticaria: a multi-centre randomized double-blind study. *Br J Dermatol* **117**:81–8.

7. Aymard JP, Lederlin P, Witz F, Colomb JN, Herbeuval R, Weber B. (1980). Cimetidine for pruritus in Hodgkin's disease. *Br Med J* **280**:151–2.

8. Weick JK, Donovan PB, Najean Y, Dresch C, Pisciotta AV, Cooperberg AA, Goldberg JD. (1982). The use of cimetidine for the treatment of pruritus in polycythemia vera. *Arch Intern Med* **142**:241–2.

9. Martinez C, Albet C, Agundez JA, Herrero E, Carrillo JA, Marquez M, Benitez J, Ortiz JA. (1999). Comparative *in vitro* and *in vivo* inhibition of cytochrome P450 CYP1A2, CYP2D6, and CYP3A by H2-receptor antagonists. *Clin Pharmacol Ther* **65**:369–76.

10. Richelson E. (1983). Antimuscarinic and other receptor-blocking properties of antidepressants. *Mayo Clin Proc* **58**:40–6.

11. Figueiredo A, Ribeiro CA, Goncalo M, Almeida L, Poiares-Baptista A, Teixeira F. (1990). Mechanism of action of doxepin in the treatment of chronic urticaria. *Fundam Clin Pharmacol* **4**:147–58.

12. Figge J, Leonard P, Richelson E. (1979). Tricyclic antidepressants: potent blockade of histamine H1 receptors of guinea pig ileum. *Eur J Pharmacol* **58**: 479–83.

13. Sabroe RA, Kennedy CT, Archer CB. (1997). The effects of topical doxepin on responses to histamine, substance P and prostaglandin E2 in human skin. *Br J Dermatol* **137**:386–90.

14. Drake LA, Fallon JD, Sober A. (1994). Relief of pruritus in patients with atopic dermatitis after treatment with topical doxepin cream. The Doxepin Study Group. *J Am Acad Dermatol* **31**:613–16.

15. Breneman D, Dunlap E, Monroe E, *et al.* (1997). Doxepin cream relieves eczema-associated pruritus within 15 minutes and is not accompanied by a risk of rebound upon discontinuation [abstract]. *J Dermatol Treat* **8**:161–8.

16. Anonymous (2000). Doxepin cream for eczema? *Drug Ther Bull* **38**:31–2.

17. Smith PF, Corelli RL. (1997). Doxepin in the management of pruritus associated with allergic cutaneous reactions. *Ann Pharmacother* **31**:633–5.

18. Borgeat A, Stirnemann HR. (1999). Ondansetron is effective to treat spinal or epidural morphine-induced pruritus. *Anesthesiology* **90**:432–6.

19. Raderer M, Muller C, Scheithauer W. (1994). Ondansetron for pruritus due to cholestasis. *N Engl J Med* **330**:1540.

20. Schworer H, Ramadori G. (1993). Improvement of cholestatic pruritus by ondansetron. *Lancet* **341**:1277.

21. Quigley C, Plowman PN. (1996). 5HT$_3$ receptor antagonists and pruritus due to cholestasis. *Palliative Med* **10**:54.

22. Balaskas EV, Bamihas GI, Karamouzis M, Voyiatzis G, Tourkantonis A. (1998). Histamine and serotonin in uremic pruritus: effect of ondansetron in CAPD-pruritic patients. *Nephron* **78**:395–402.

23. O'Donohue JW, Haigh C, Williams R. (1997). Ondansetron in the treatment of pruritus of cholestasis: a randomised controlled trial. *Gastroenterology* **112**:A1349.

24. Muller C, Pongratz S, Pidlich J, Penner E, Kaider A, Schemper M, Raderer M, Scheithauer W, Ferenci P. (1998). Treatment of pruritus in chronic liver disease with the 5-hydroxytryptamine receptor type 3 antagonist ondansetron: a randomized, placebo-controlled, double-blind cross-over trial. *Eur J Gastroenterol Hepatol* **10**:865–70.

25. Murphy M, Reich D, Pai P, Finn P, Carmichael AJ. (2003). A randomized, placebo-controlled, double-blind trial of ondansetron in renal itch. *Br J Dermatol* **148**:314–17.

26. Zylicz Z, Smits C, Krajnik M. (1998). Paroxetine for pruritus in advanced cancer. *J Pain Symptom Manage* **16**:121–4.

27. Diehn F, Tefferi A. (2001). Pruritus in polycythaemia vera: prevalence, laboratory correlates and management. *Br J Haematol* **115**:619–21.

28. Tefferi A, Fonseca R. (2002). Selective serotonin reuptake inhibitors are effective in the treatment of polycythemia vera-associated pruritus. *Blood* **99**:2627.

29. de Boer T. (1995). The effects of mirtazapine on central noradrenergic and serotonergic neurotransmission. *Int Clin Psychopharmacol* **10** (Suppl. 4):19–23.

30. Clough GF, Boutsiouki P, Church MK. (2001). Comparison of the effects of levocetirizine and loratadine on histamine- induced wheal, flare, and itch in human skin. *Allergy* **56**:985–8.

31. Davis MP, Frandsen JL, Walsh D, Andresen S, Taylor S. (2003). Mirtazapine for pruritus. *J Pain Symptom Manage* **25**:288–91.

32. Metze D, Reimann S, Beissert S, Luger T. (1999). Efficacy and safety of naltrexone, an oral opiate receptor antagonist, in the treatment of pruritus in internal and dermatological diseases. *J Am Acad Dermatol* **41**:533–9.

33. Bergasa NV, Talbot TL, Alling DW, Schmitt JM, Walker EC, Baker BL, Korenman JC, Park Y, Hoofnagle JH, Jones EA. (1992). A controlled trial of naloxone infusions for the pruritus of chronic cholestasis. *Gastroenterology* **102**:544–9.

34. Bergasa NV, Alling DW, Talbot TL, Swain MG, Yurdaydin C, Turner ML, Schmitt JM, Walker EC, Jones EA. (1995). Effects of naloxone infusions in patients with the pruritus of cholestasis. A double-blind, randomized, controlled trial. *Ann Intern Med* **123**:161–7.

35. Basnet P, Yasuda I, Kumagai N, Tohda C, Nojima H, Kuraishi Y, Komatsu K. (2001). Inhibition of itch–scratch response by fruits of *Cnidium monnieri* in mice. *Biol Pharm Bull* **24**:1012–5.

36. Bergasa NV, Schmitt JM, Talbot TL, Alling DW, Swain MG, Turner ML, Jenkins JB, Jones EA. (1998). Open-label trial of oral nalmefene therapy for the pruritus of cholestasis. *Hepatology* **27**:679–84.

37. Bergasa NV, Alling DW, Talbot TL, Wells MC, Jones EA. (1999). Oral nalmefene therapy reduces scratching activity due to the pruritus of cholestasis: a controlled study. *J Am Acad Dermatol* **41**:431–4.

38. Picard D, Jousson O. (2001). Genetic variability among cercariae of the Schistosomatidae (Trematoda: Digenea) causing swimmer's itch in Europe. *Parasite* **8**:237–42.

39. Carson KL, Tran TT, Cotton P, Sharara AI, Hunt CM. (1996). Pilot study of the use of naltrexone to treat the severe pruritus of cholestatic liver disease. *Am J Gastroenterol* **91**:1022–3.

40. Wolfhagen FH, Sternieri E, Hop WC, Vitale G, Bertolotti M, Van Buuren HR. (1997). Oral naltrexone treatment for cholestatic pruritus: a double-blind, placebo-controlled study. *Gastroenterology* **113**:1264–9.

41. Sakai T, Fukano T, Sumikawa K. (2001). IV butorphanol reduces analgesia but not pruritus or nausea associated with intrathecal morphine. *Can J Anaesth* **48**:831–2.

42. Thornton JR, Losowsky MS. (1988). Opioid peptides and primary biliary cirrhosis. *Br Med J* **297**:1501–4.

43. Jones EA, Dekker LR. (2000). Florid opioid withdrawal-like reaction precipitated by naltrexone in a patient with chronic cholestasis. *Gastroenterology* **118**:431–2.

44. Jones EA, Neuberger J, Bergasa NV. (2002). Opiate antagonist therapy for the pruritus of cholestasis: the avoidance of opioid withdrawal-like reactions. *QJM* **95**:547–52.

45. Ponnighaus JM, Ziegler H, Suckow M, Kowalzick L. (2000). Pruritus of dark skin in hookworm infection [in German]. *Hautarzt* **51**:953–5.

46. Mitchell JE. (1986). Naltrexone and hepatotoxicity. *Lancet* **1**:1215.

47. Juby LD, Wong VS, Losowsky MS. (1994). Buprenorphine and hepatic pruritus. *Br J Clin Pract* **48**:331.

48. Zylicz Z, Krajnik M. (1999). Codeine for pruritus in primary billiary cirrhosis. *Lancet* **353**:813.

49. Ghent CN, Carruthers SG. (1988). Treatment of pruritus in primary biliary cirrhosis with rifampin. Results of a double-blind, crossover, randomized trial. *Gastroenterology* **94**:488–93.

50. Anwer MS, Kroker R, Hegner D. (1978). Inhibition of hepatic uptake of bile acids by rifamycins. *Naunyn Schmiedebergs Arch Pharmacol* **302**:19–24.

51. Bachs L, Pares A, Elena M, Piera C, Rodes J. (1989). Comparison of rifampicin with phenobarbitone for treatment of pruritus in biliary cirrhosis. *Lancet* **1**:574–6.

52. Bloomer JR, Boyer JL. (1975). Phenobarbital effects in cholestatic liver diseases. *Ann Intern Med* **82**:310–17.

53. Sharp HL, Carey JB Jr, White JG, Krivit W. (1967). Cholestyramine therapy in patients with a paucity of intrahepatic bile ducts. *J Pediatr* **71**:723–36.

54. Datta DV, Sherlock S. (1966). Cholestyramine for long term relief of the pruritus complicating intrahepatic cholestasis. *Gastroenterology* **50**:323–32.

55. Ahrens E, Payne M, Kunkel H. (1950). Primary biliry cirrhosis. *Medicine* **29**: 299–364.

56. Lloyd-Thomas H, Sherlock S. (1952). Testosterone therapy for the pruritus of obstructive jaundice. *Br Med J* **ii**:1289–91.

57. Welder AA, Robertson JW, Melchert RB. (1995). Toxic effects of anabolic–androgenic steroids in primary rat hepatic cell cultures. *J Pharmacol Toxicol Methods* **33**:187–95.

58. Bergasa NV, Sabol SL, Young WS 3rd, Kleiner DE, Jones EA. (1995). Cholestasis is associated with preproenkephalin mRNA expression in the adult rat liver. *Am J Physiol* **268**:G346–54.

59. Gurakar A, Caraceni P, Fagiuoli S, Van Thiel DH. (1994). Androgenic/anabolic steroid-induced intrahepatic cholestasis: a review with four additional case reports. *J Okla State Med Assoc* **87**:399–404.

60. Massry SG, Popovtzer MM, Coburn JW, Makoff DL, Maxwell MH, Kleeman CR. (1968). Intractable pruritus as a manifestation of secondary hyperparathyroidism in uremia. Disappearance of itching after subtotal parathyroidectomy. *N Engl J Med* **279**:697–700.

61. Gilchrest BA, Rowe JW, Brown RS, Steinman TI, Arndt KA. (1979). Ultraviolet phototherapy of uremic pruritus. Long-term results and possible mechanism of action. *Ann Intern Med* **91**:17–21.

62. Blachley JD, Blankenship DM, Menter A, Parker TF 3d, Knochel JP. (1985). Uremic pruritus: skin divalent ion content and response to ultraviolet phototherapy. *Am J Kidney Dis* **5**:237–41.

63. Peer G, Kivity S, Agami O, *et al.* (1996). Randomised crossover trial of naltrexone in uraemic pruritus. *Lancet* **348**:1552–4.

64. Pauli-Magnus C, Mikus G, Alscher DM, *et al.* (2000). Naltrexone does not relieve uremic pruritus: results of a randomized, double-blind, placebo-controlled crossover study. *J Am Soc Nephrol* 11:514–19.

65. Silva SR, Viana PC, Lugon NV, Hoette M, Ruzany F, Lugon JR. (1994). Thalidomide for the treatment of uremic pruritus: a crossover randomized double-blind trial. *Nephron* 67:270–3.

66. Finelli C, Gugliotta L, Gamberi B, Vianelli N, Visani G, Tura S. (1993). Relief of intractable pruritus in polycythemia vera with recombinant interferon alfa. *Am J Hematol* 43:316–18.

67. Muller EW, de Wolf JT, Egger R, *et al.* (1995). Long-term treatment with interferon-alpha 2b for severe pruritus in patients with polycythaemia vera. *Br J Haematol* 89 :313–18.

68. Fjellner B, Hägermark O. (1979). Pruritus in polycythemia vera: treatment with aspirin and possibility of platelet involvement. *Acta Derm Venereol* 59:505–12.

69. Jackson N, Burt D, Crocker J, Boughton B. (1987). Skin mast cells in poly-cythaemia vera: relationship to the pathogenesis and treatment of pruritus. *Br J Dermatol* 116:21–9.

70. Morgan PW, Berridge JC. (2000). Giving long-persistent starch as volume replacement can cause pruritus after cardiac surgery. *Br J Anaesth* 85:696–9.

71. Gobbi PG, Attardo-Parrinello G, Lattanzio G, Rizzo SC, Ascari E. (1983). Severe pruritus should be a B-symptom in Hodgkin's disease. *Cancer* 51:1934–6.

72. Cockerell C. (1994). The itches of HIV infection and AIDS. In: Bernhard, J. (ed.), *Itch, mechanisms and management of pruritus*, New York: McGraw-Hill, pp. 347–65.

73. Smith KJ, Skelton HG, Yeager J, Lee RB, Wagner KF. (1997). Pruritus in HIV-1 disease: therapy with drugs which may modulate the pattern of immune dysregulation. *Dermatology* 195:353–8.

74. Asokumar B, Newman LM, McCarthy RJ, Ivankovich AD, Tuman KJ. (1998). Intrathecal bupivacaine reduces pruritus and prolongs duration of fentanyl analgesia during labor: a prospective, randomized controlled trial. *Anesth Analg* 87:1309–15.

75. Korbon G, James D, Verlander J. (1985). Intramuscular naloxone reverses the side effects of epidural morphine while preserving analgesia. *Regional Anaesthesia* 10:16–20.

76. Ueyama H, Nishimura M, Tashiro C. (1992). Naloxone reversal of nystagmus associated with intrathecal morphine administration. *Anesthesiology* 76:153.

77. Pierard GE, Henry F, Pierard-Franchimont C. (2000). Pharma-clinics. How I treat . . . pruritus by an antihistamine [in French]. *Rev Med Liege* 55:763–6.

78. Kjellberg F, Tramer MR. (2001). Pharmacological control of opioid-induced pruritus: a quantitative systematic review of randomized trials. *Eur J Anaesthesiol* 18:346–57.

79. Cohen SE, Ratner EF, Kreitzman TR, Archer JH, Mignano LR. (1992). Nalbuphine is better than naloxone for treatment of side effects after epidural morphine. *Anesth Analg* **75**:747–52.

80. Dunteman E, Karanikolas M, Filos KS. (1996). Transnasal butorphanol for the treatment of opioid-induced pruritus unresponsive to antihistamines. *J Pain Symptom Manage* **12**:255–60.

81. Gunter JB, McAuliffe J, Gregg T, Weidner N, Varughese AM, Sweeney DM. (2000). Continuous epidural butorphanol relieves pruritus associated with epidural morphine infusions in children. *Paediatr Anaesth* **10**:167–72.

82. Franco J. (1999). Pruritus. *Curr Treat Options Gastroenterol* **2**:451–6.

83. Bernstein JE, Grinzi RA. (1981). Butorphanol-induced pruritus antagonized by naloxone. *J Am Acad Dermatol* **5**:227–8.

84. Borgeat A, Wilder-Smith OH, Saiah M, Rifat K. (1992). Subhypnotic doses of propofol relieve pruritus induced by epidural and intrathecal morphine. *Anesthesiology* **76**:510–12.

85. Colbert S, O'Hanlon DM, Chambers F, Moriarty DC. (1999). The effect of intravenous tenoxicam on pruritus in patients receiving epidural fentanyl. *Anaesthesia* **54**:76–80.

86. Colbert S, O'Hanlon DM, Galvin S, Chambers F, Moriarty DC. (1999). The effect of rectal diclofenac on pruritus in patients receiving intrathecal morphine. *Anaesthesia* **54**:948–52.

87. Katcher J, Walsh D. (1999). Opioid-induced itching: morphine sulfate and hydromorphone hydrochloride. *J Pain Symptom Manage* **17**:70–2.

14

Treatment of patients with pruritus from the nursing perspective

Harmieke van Os and Petra Eland

Pruritus and the quality of life

Pruritus is a major symptom of many skin diseases and systemic non-skin diseases. Despite this, it remains poorly studied in relation to its pathophysiology and treatment, as well in terms of its impact on the patient's daily life.[1–3] Pruritus causes the patient considerable distress and affects quality of life.[4, 5]

Itching is commonly defined as a sensation that provokes the desire to scratch.[3, 6] Therefore scratching is a behavioural response. The vicious itch–scratch cycle is frequently a consequence of itching and scratching. This vicious cycle is always present in atopic dermatitis[7] and is also seen in other skin disorders. The pruritus is often so distressing that patients scratch themselves until they bleed. Scratching stops itching in the short term and leads to a decreased pruritus threshold once the skin starts to heal.[7] Scratching stops itching for a while but also leads to a greater secretion of inflammation mediators, which exacerbates the itching and reinforces the cycle.[8]

Sleep disturbances in atopic dermatitis are often associated with itching and scratching.[9] This is possibly because pruritus that is not caused by psychogenic factors occurs mainly during the evening and at night.[5, 8] In a study with 101 patients with psoriasis, 84% of the patients experienced generalized pruritus.[5] In about two-thirds of patients pruritus was associated with difficulty falling asleep and the same proportion was awakened by the pruritus. When pruritus interferes with sleep, it also impairs performance at school and work.[10] Patients often become more agitated and tired.

When in contact with others, especially with spouses or family members, itching and scratching may cause anger and resentment. Patients with pruritus often mention their partner's intolerance of scratching.[11] The constant scratching and the resultant physical disfigurement may lead to feelings of shame and diminished self-esteem.[10, 11]

Influence of emotional stress, anxiety, and depression

The most important pruritic skin disorders that are recognized as having a psychosomatic component are psoriasis, atopic eczema, and chronic idiopathic urticaria (see Chapter 11). Emotional stress has been observed to exacerbate or affect the course of these skin disorders.[6] Other psychological factors affecting especially atopic dermatitis are major and minor life events, daily hassles, and stressful communication with others.[7] Two psychological symptoms—anxiety and depression—have been investigated in pruritis patients. These symptoms appear to be frequent concomitants of pruritic dermatoses. However, it is impossible to say with certainty whether pruritus is a result of anxiety or depression or whether the observed incidence of anxiety or depression merely represents a reaction to a persistent and distressing symptom.[6, 8, 12–14]

Nursing interventions in coping with pruritus

Pruritus is a multidisciplinary and complex problem that has a lot of consequences for patients in their daily lives. The prescribed treatment does not automatically lead to success. Nursing interventions are based on problems that occur as a result of itching and scratching.

Daily skin care

A common cause of pruritus is dry skin (xerosis).[15, 16] Dry skin is often present in a skin disease such as atopic dermatitis.[17] A dry skin can also be caused by frequent use of water and soap, or by ageing processes in skin.[16]

To minimize xerosis-associated pruritus, bathing in lukewarm water is preferable and should be limited to 10 minutes.[18] Hot water increases histamine release and histamine is an important mediator of certain types of pruritus.[8] Gentle cleansing agents should be used: "abrasive" soaps can cause irritation, and even inflammation of the skin, whereas bath oils are often comforting.[18] After bathing the skin should be carefully dabbed dry, and emollient applied.[15, 16, 18, 19] Emollients contain various amounts of water and lipids, and have different consistencies and degrees of oiliness.[17] Creams spread easily on the skin but are soaked up quickly when the skin is very dry. Ointments have a more oily mixture and tend to be greasier, therefore giving an occlusive effect and retaining water in the skin. Emollients have an antipruritic effect, although the exact antipruritic mechanism is not fully understood.[17] In one-third of the patients with psoriasis surveyed, itching, soreness, redness, scaling, and extension of lesions were reduced by twice-daily application of emollients.[20] A regime of applying emollients twice-daily requires time and effort by patients and their families. To achieve compliance, the following factors must be taken into account when choosing an emollient:

• the patient's individual preference;

• the emollient's consistency;

• care must be taken to avoid ingredients that could cause problems for the patient, such as fragrances, preservatives, or lanolin.[17]

Recognizing and avoiding triggering factors

Water and soap may trigger pruritus. However, there are additional factors that can aggravate pruritus, for example, warmth, perspiration, wool, nutrition, alcohol, dry air, and physical condition.[15, 21, 22] Recognizing and avoiding these factors is part of the art of treating pruritus.[10]

Warmth and perspiration stimulate the C-fibres, probably causing pruritus.[8] To avoid irritations through perspiration advise the patient to take a short lukewarm shower and apply an emollient after sporting activities. It is also wise to avoid very warm surroundings and to try to minimize sweating.[15] A cool and well-ventilated living environment is preferable. Wool can irritate the skin; therefore it is recommended to avoid woollen clothes and blankets. Anything that increases blood flow through the skin, such as heat, alcohol, hot and spicy food, and febrile illness, is more likely to generate itching in patients with atopic dermatitis.[10] Dry air caused in winter by indoor heating and by air conditioning in hot summers is another trigger. Ambient humidity can be maintained by placing a cool-mist vaporizer in the room.[18] Cooling the skin can give pruritus relief by directly inhibiting cutaneous itch receptors. Cool compresses, cool baths or showers, or cool moist air may be helpful.[10, 15, 18] Another way to cool the skin is by using menthol. Menthol can be added to emollients, medical ointments, or creams. Menthol acts on the cold receptors of the skin to cause a feeling of coolness.[16, 18]

Awareness training and habit reversal

One of the major problems for patients with pruritus is scratching. The cycle of itching and scratching occurs frequently. 'Automatic' scratching is also a recognized phenomenon. An example would be scratching due to tension or habit that occurs without prior itching.[7] Reduction of scratching activity and breaking the itch–scratch cycle are important goals in the treatment of skin diseases.[8, 22–24]

A commonly used intervention to reduce scratching is habit reversal. This intervention was developed in 1974 and was reviewed by Miltenberger *et al.*[25] Habit reversal comprises four phases:

1. Awareness training. This is used to enable the patient to distinguish between the occurrence of itching and scratching. A diary is often used to increase patients' awareness.

2. Competing response training. The patient uses a competing response (incompatible behaviour) for 3 minutes during the occurrence of the habit or awareness that the habit is about to occur. Incompatible behaviour is, for example, clenching one's fists or turning a ring on one's finger.

3. Motivation phase. This phase involves three procedures: reviewing all the situations in which the habit was inconvenient or embarrassing; social support training to instruct others to prompt the patient to use the competing response; and practising the competing response in situations in which the habit is likely to occur.

4. Generalization procedure. The competing response is used in all relevant situations and social support is used to promote a successful outcome.

The results of studies of the effectiveness of habit reversal are encouraging. Rosenbaum and Ayllon[26] treated four patients with atopic dermatitis with habit reversal. They concluded that, using this method, scratching decreased over a period of 6 months. Melin *et al.*[27] compared, in a randomized controlled study, the use of habit reversal in combination with a hydrocortisone cream with the use of cream alone in a group of 17 patients with atopic dermatitis. There was significantly more improvement in the skin lesions in the group that received habit reversal than in the control group.

Habit reversal often constitutes a part of a combined treatment. Ehlers *et al.*[7] compared the effectiveness of treatment for atopic dermatitis in a randomized controlled study in which there were four treatment groups.

Patients who received a combined dermatological and behavioural programme exhibited larger reductions in frequency of itching and scratching than patients in the other groups. In this study habit reversal was part of the behavioural treatment. Patients receiving relaxation therapy, behavioural treatment, or a combination of these approaches exhibited significantly larger decreases in itching than patients receiving standard medical care. Encouraging results of awareness training and habit reversal in combination with psychotherapy are also described in case studies.[28, 29]

Stress management and relaxation exercises

Stress may increase pruritus and exacerbate dermatological diseases such as atopic dermatitis and psoriasis. Stress can also be a consequence of pruritus. Therefore, stress management (e.g. assertiveness training and cognitive therapy) and relaxation exercises are often part of a behavioural treatment programme for patients with atopic eczema.[7, 23, 30] Van Rood and Ouwehand[31] suggest the use of relaxation training when stress is a result of physical symptoms or when physical symptoms are sustained by stress. Relaxation training may also be helpful when a patient experiences stress due to sleep disturbances, medical investigations, or treatment. Psychological intervention, such as stress management and relaxation exercises, may lead to a significant improvement of skin lesions, scratching frequency, and self-reported indices of distress.[7, 30] Patient self-management may also be improved by a combination of psycho-educational and dermatological treatment.[9] Stress decreases in psoriatic patients who receive individual psychotherapy that includes stress management and relaxation.[32] In the evaluation of a programme of sessions about psoriasis, feelings of acceptance, stress management, and coping with daily life, patients reported an enhanced knowledge about psoriasis and an increase of coping skills and self-confidence.[9, 33]

Patient advocacy groups may be beneficial in improving quality of life. They offer patient education at meetings and provide support brochures. They can also address and correct common patient myths about disease and its treatment and offer emotional support.[34]

Patient education and compliance

Patients' compliance with the medical or nursing interventions is necessary to achieve successful outcomes. It is a frequent issue of concern in the treatment of skin diseases.[23] Compliance requires the confidence and cooperation of the patient, the patient's family, and non-professional care-givers.[34, 35] Health education, health promotion, and counselling are used to ensure better cooperation and understanding by the patient. Patients with psoriasis, for example, have to be educated in such a way that they understand certain information about their skin condition, in particular, that it is a chronic problem and that (rapid) cure is not to be expected. Thus the patient will not be disappointed when the desired effects of treatment are not immediate.[36] Kalimo *et al.*[37] studied the benefit of a nurse-led education programme to improve treatment compliance and skin protection. In this programme the nurse discusses all aspects of treatment, protection, and avoidance of allergens with patients with occupational skin disease. The results suggest that the outcome of dermatitis can be influenced favourably by active patient cooperation and individual consultations with a trained nurse. Poor adherence to therapy may occur with the use of corticosteroids. Charman *et al.*[38] emphasize the need to provide patients with atopic dermatitis with information and education regarding the safety, potency, and appropriate use of topical corticosteroids. They expected that better education could improve patients' compliance. Their study suggested an irrational fear of topical corticosteroids; 72.5% of the patients are worried about the use of these drugs, whereas concern about the use of emollients does not seem to be a common problem. Because of their concerns 24% of patients did not use the topical corticosteroids. Thus, their concerns affected compliance. In general, patient education is an important (nursing) intervention to increase patient self-management in coping with diseases or handicaps.[19, 23, 38, 39] Other effects of patient education include increasing patients' knowledge and skills and reduction of anxiety.[39] Patient education may consist of provision of information (e.g. information about pruritus), instruction (e.g. about how to use emollients), education (e.g. awareness training), and psychosocial support.[40] Health and medical workers need to provide patients with information about their diagnosis and treatment since it is the patients' legal right.[39]

Terra *et al.*[39] have developed a model for patient education based on a behavioural perspective. Behavioural change can be approached through patient education. In this context the following points are relevant. The patient must be:

• responsive to new information;

• able to understand what he or she is told;

• willing to change his or her behaviour;

- capable of acquiring new skills;
- willing to put the newly learned skills into practice.
- able to accept that the new behaviour has a place in his/her daily life.

To achieve a satisfactory behavioural change, it is necessary that all of these requirements are met. Behavioural changes and overall outcome will be influenced only by taking into account the patient's personal situation, coping strategies, attitude, and social support. Essential elements in this approach are verbal and written information, practical exercises, modelling, counselling, and social resources.

The pruritus treatment programme 'Coping with itch'

The treatment programme, 'Coping with itch', for patients with pruritus has been developed in the Netherlands, based on the interventions described above.[40] This programme is carried out in sessions for patients with skin-disease-induced pruritus. Nurses at an out-patient department of dermatology supervise these individual consulting sessions. The central purpose of these sessions is to help the patient cope with his or her pruritus. The nursing consultation is in addition to the standard medical treatment by the dermatologist; patients are referred to this programme by dermatologists. Consulting sessions are delivered individually on the premise that the patient's perspective and individual problems accompanying the itching and scratching in his or her daily life are the beginning of the treatment. The programme consists of three or four sessions lasting 45 minutes over an average of 4 months. Nurses lead the sessions because the most important task for a nurse is to help patients to cope with their chronic (skin) disease in daily life.[41] Nurses at an out-patient department of dermatology are part of a multidisciplinary team with dermatologists and medical social workers and psychologists. It is possible to refer to one of the other members of the team when necessary. Interventions of the programme 'Coping with itch' are described in the following section.

The essentials of the programme 'Coping with itch'

The consulting sessions start with the introduction in which patient's expectations and cooperation are discussed. Next, a pruritus history is taken to understand the patient's viewpoint, needs, and perception of disease.[40] The pruritus history consists of questions on the following topics.

- The skin disease. Which skin disease do you have and which medical treatment do you receive?
- Itching and scratching. At what times of the day does the pruritus occur?
- Which factors affect itching (physical, psychological, environmental); when and how do you scratch?
- Relationship to food, menstruation cycle, and sleep.
- Coping with itch and skin hygiene. Questions include which skin care is used; the use of soap, emollients, or other products; product preferences; compliance with prescribed treatment.
- The meaning of pruritus for the patient. The effects on his or her life, moods, relationships, and work and does it disturb sleep.

The history is completed by a thorough inspection of the skin. A care strategy is proposed to the patient.

Patient education is an important intervention in the 'Coping with itch' programme. Attention is given to:

- the phenomenon of pruritus, its effects, and standard medical treatment;
- patient advocacy groups;
- coping with triggering factors of pruritus: the use of cold in relieving pruritus, daily skin care and protection, preventing damage by scratching;
- compliance with the prescribed treatment of the skin disease, and of the itching and scratching, for example, the use of emollients, medicinal creams, ointments, and oral medications, and the undesirable effects of the medical treatment;
- coping with an acute exacerbation and the support of health professionals or family;
- awareness training.

In addition, to help patients become aware of the frequency and intensity of itching and scratching, the circumstances, and the measures taken to relieve the pruritus, it is useful to keep an 'itch diary'. Patients should keep a diary for 7 days, after which the nurse will discuss the diary. During the discussion patients discover at which times during the day itching usually occurs, the occurrence of automatic scratching, the influence of stress on the intensity of itch, and the effect of measures taken to relieve itch. Patients' brochures support all verbal information and instructions.

Another intervention in the programme 'Coping with itch' is psychosocial support. Nurses have to be alert to psychosocial problems, but also to patients' skills and capacities to cope with these problems. Psychosocial support consists of helping to analyse problems and to deal with daily hassles, and giving encouragement to patients. Thereby the confidence and cooperation of the patient and his family members are ensured.[41] More specific interventions include the following.

1. Habit reversal. Awareness training using an itch diary is often the first step of the habit reversal programme. To participate in the habit reversal programme three conditions have to be fulfilled.

   • The patient himself wants to diminish scratching.
   • The patient recognizes that the itch–scratch cycle occurs.
   • The patient recognizes automatic scratching.

   The details of the habit reversal were given earlier in this chapter. Patient information brochures have been developed for the itch diary and habit reversal.

2. Relaxation exercises. Relaxation exercises are indicated in cases of stress due to itching, sleep disturbances, or as a form of diversion. The nurse gives the patient instruction in progressive muscle relaxation or suggestive relaxation in which a slow and heavy sensation is suggested. Patients have to practise this exercise once or twice daily, with the help of a cassette tape with verbal instructions.

3. Referral. The nurse can refer patients to a medical social worker or psychologist if there are relationship problems, work-related problems, or other problems. The nurse refers to a dermatologist for medical problems. It is important to inform patients of the reason for the referral.

Conclusions

• Care for patients with pruritus is a multidisciplinary problem and nursing interventions are an important aspect of this care.

• Information and motivation of the patient are paramount.

• Learning to avoid factors that provoke pruritus is the first step to changing of behaviour.

• Awareness of scratching can be easily brought to the fore with a diary.

• Programmes such as 'Coping with itch' that aim to achieve habit reversal have the potential of improving patients' quality of life and can be an important contribution to the overall treatment.

References

1. Gupta MA, Gupta AK, Schork NJ, Ellis CN. (1994). Depression modulates pruritus perception: a study of pruritus in psoriasis, atopic dermatitis, and chronic idiopathic urticaria. *Psychosom Med* **56**:36–40.

2. Greaves MW. (1997). Anti-itch treatments: do they work? *Skin Pharmacol* **10**:225–9.

3. Rees JL, Laidlaw A. (1999). Pruritus: more scratch than itch. *Clin Exp Dermatol* **24**:490–3.

4. Kam PC, Tan KH. (1996). Pruritus—itching for a cause and relief? *Anaesthesia* **51**:1133–8.

5. Yosipovitch G, Goon A, Wee J, Chan YH, Goh CL. (2000). The prevalence and clinical characteristics of pruritus among patients with extensive psoriasis. *Br J Dermatol* **143**:969–73.

6. Gupta MA, Gupta AK. (1999). Depression modulates pruritus perception. A study of pruritus in psoriasis, atopic dermatitis and chronic idiopathic urticaria. *Ann NY Acad Sci* **885**:394–5.

7. Ehlers A, Stangier U, Gieler U. (1995). Treatment of atopic dermatitis: a comparison of psychological and dermatological approaches to relapse prevention. *J Consult Clin Psychol* **63**:624–35.

8. Yosipovitch G, David M. (1999). The diagnostic and therapeutic approach to idiopathic generalized pruritus. *Int J Dermatol* **38**:881–7.

9. Jaspers JPC, Span L, Molier L, Coenraads PJ. (2000). A multimodal education and treatment programme for young adults with atopic dermatitis: a randomised controlled trial. *Dermatol Psychosom* **1**:148–53.

10. Koblenzer CS. (1999). Itching and the atopic skin. *J Allergy Clin Immunol* **104**:S109–13.

11. Jowett S, Ryan T. (1985). Skin disease and handicap: an analysis of the impact of skin conditions. *Soc Sci Med* **20**:425–9.

12. Gupta MA, Gupta AK, Kirkby S, *et al.* (1988). Pruritus in psoriasis. A prospective study of some psychiatric and dermatologic correlates. *Arch Dermatol* **124**:1052–7.

13. Sheehan-Dare RA, Henderson MJ, Cotterill JA. (1990). Anxiety and depression in patients with chronic urticaria and generalized pruritus. *Br J Dermatol* **123**:769–74.

14. Radmanesh M, Shafiei S. (2001). Underlying psychopathologies of psychogenic pruritic disorders. *Dermatol Psychosom* **2**:130–1.

15. Hägermark O, Wahlgren CF. (1995). Treatment of itch. *Semin Dermatol* **14**:320–5.

16. Fleischer AB Jr. (1995). Pruritus in the elderly. *Adv Dermatol* **10**:41–59.

17. Burr S. (1999). Emollients for managing dry skin conditions. *Prof Nurse* **15**:43–8.

18. Bueller HA, Bernhard JD. (1998). Review of pruritus therapy. *Dermatol Nurs* **10**:101–7.

19. Bernhard JD. (1994). General principles, overview and miscellaneous treatments of itching. In: Bernhard JD. (ed.), *Itch, mechanisms and management of pruritus*, New York: McGraw-Hill, pp. 367–81.

20. Greaves MW, Weinstein GD. (1995). Treatment of psoriasis. *N Engl J Med* **332**:581–8.

21. Wahlgren CF. (1991). Itch and atopic dermatitis: clinical and experimental studies. *Acta Derm Venereol Suppl (Stockh)* **165**:1–53.

22. Lawton S. (1996). Living with eczema: the dermatology patient. *Br J Nurs* **5**:600–4, 606–9.

23. Jaspers JPC. (1994). Behavioural therapy in patients with chronic skin disease. *Clin Psychol Psychiatry* **1**:202–9.

24. Beltrani VS. (1999). Managing atopic dermatitis. *Dermatol Nurs* **11**:171–6.

25. Miltenberger RG, Fuqua RW, Woods DW. (1998). Applying behavior analysis to clinical problems: review and analysis of habit reversal. *J Appl Behav Anal* **31**:447–69.

26. Rosenbaum MS, Ayllon T. (1981). The behavioral treatment of neurodermatitis through habit-reversal. *Behav Res Ther* **19**:313–18.

27. Melin L, Frederiksen T, Noren P, Swebilius BG. (1986). Behavioural treatment of scratching in patients with atopic dermatitis. *Br J Dermatol* **115**:467–74.

28. Nabarro G. (1995). Psychotherapie bij atopisch eczeem [in Dutch]. *Ned Tijdschr Dermatol Venereol* **5**:206–8.

29. van der Schaar WW, Lamberts H. (1997). Scratching for the itch in eczema; a psychodermatologic approach [in Dutch]. *Ned Tijdschr Geneeskd* **141**:2049–51.

30. Cole WC, Roth HL, Sachs LB. (1988). Group psychotherapy as an aid in the medical treatment of eczema. *J Am Acad Dermatol* **18**:286–91.

31. van Rood YR, Ouwehand A. (2001). Het gebruik van ontspanningsoefeningen bij patienten die zijn opgenomen voor een somatische aandoening [in Dutch]. *Directieve Therapie* **21**:147–58.

32. Zachariae R, Oster H, Bjerring P, Kragballe K. (1996). Effects of psychologic intervention on psoriasis: a preliminary report. *J Am Acad Dermatol* **34**:1008–15.

33. Tan KS, Tham SN. (1997). Group therapy: a useful and supportive treatment for psoriasis patients. *Int J Dermatol* **36**:110–12.

34. Rolstad T, Zimmerman G. (2000). Patient advocacy groups. A key prescription for dermatology. *Dermatol Clin* **18**:277–85.

35. Dennis H, Watts J. (1998). Skin care in atopic eczema. *Professional Nurse* **13**:s10–s13.

36. Watts J. (1999). Update psoriasis. *Professional Nurse* **14**:623–6.

37. Kalimo K, Kautiainen H, Niskanen T, Niemi L. (1999). 'Eczema school' to improve compliance in an occupational dermatology clinic. *Contact Dermatitis* **41**:315–19.

38. Charman CR, Morris AD, Williams HC. (2000). Topical corticosteroid phobia in patients with atopic eczema. *Br J Dermatol* **142**:931–6.

39. Terra B, Mechelen-Gevers E, Williams HC, van den Burgt M. (2000). *Doen wat kan, patiëntenvoorlichting door verpleegkundigen* [in Dutch]. Maarssen: Elsevier Gezondheidszorg.

40. Eland-de Kok PCM, Os-Medendorp H. (1999). Huidproblemen (jeuk) [in Dutch]. In: van Achterberg T, Eliens AM, Strijdbol NCM. (eds.). *Effectief verplegen*. Dwingeloo: Kavanah, pp. 195–221.

41. Johnson-Taylor E, Jones P, Burns M. (1990). Quality of life. In: Lubkin IM. (ed.), *Chronic illness: impact and intervention*, Boston: Jones and Bartlett Publishers, pp. 436–40.

15

Pruritus: past, present, and future

Robert Twycross

Transition from past to present

Although pruritus is a dominant symptom in many skin diseases and also occurs in some systemic disorders, it has never achieved 'flavour of the month' status. It is a Cinderella symptom, tucked away in a corner (like an unwanted orphan) and obscured by the glare and publicity surrounding the more fashionable members of the household, such as 'pain' and 'immunology'. So far, no one has founded the International Association for the Study of Pruritus.

Given that pruritus, like pain, is a pointer to an underlying disorder, and that cure or amelioration of the disorder will result in the resolution of the pruritus, it is understandable that physicians generally focus on identifying and treating the primary disorder rather than the secondary pruritus. However, when the causal disorder cannot be cured, patients can be left with a distressing, possibly intolerable, pruritus that significantly impairs their sense of well-being and quality of life.

The past

By this point, most physicians will have prescribed an H_1-antihistamine and turned their attention to the next patient. After all, as everybody knows (so it is said), pruritus is caused by histamine release from mast cells in the skin and is treated with topical and/or systemic H_1-antihistamines. However, if this book does little else, I hope that it will finally destroy this particular misconception.

Table 15.1 H$_1$-antihistamines

Properties	Examples
First-generation H$_1$-antihistamines Lipophilic → ready penetration of the blood–brain barrier; cause dose-dependent sedation and antimuscarinic effects, sometimes marked	Chlorphenamine, hydroxyzine, promethazine
Second-generation H$_1$-antihistamines Hydrophilic; little sedation and antimuscarinic effects	Astemizole, cetirizine, loratidine
Third-generation H$_1$-antihistamines Highly hydrophilic with very little or no sedation and antimuscarinic effects	Descarbothexyloratidine, fexofenadine, norastemizole

As noted elsewhere (see Chapter 2), histamine release plays an essential role in only a few, usually acute, conditions such as urticaria, insect bites, and drug rashes. Thus, apart from the rare condition of cutaneous mastocytosis, low-sedative second- and third-generation H$_1$-antihistamines (Table 15.1) are of little or no value in chronic pruritus associated with such disparate disorders as atopic dermatitis, psoriasis, cholestasis, uraemia, and lymphoma. In these circumstances, any benefit from a sedative first-generation H$_1$-antihistamine stems from a central effect distinct from peripheral H$_1$-receptor antagonism (Box 15.1 and Fig. 15.1).[1] Accordingly, it may be better to use a benzodiazepine in these circumstances, if only to help break the false association in the physician's mind between pruritus and histamine.

It should also be noted that not all sedatives appear to be equally beneficial. In one study, nitrazepam was compared with butobarbital in relation to impact on nocturnal pruritus.[2] Although the subjective pruritus scores were more or less identical with both drugs, the total limb movements were *increased* in patients receiving butobarbital but *decreased* when taking nitrazepam (Fig. 15.2).[2]

The present: scientific studies

Clinical observation and controlled trials, particularly over the last decade or so, have done much to aid our understanding of pruritus in liver disease (see Chapter 5) and uraemia (see Chapter 6). It is now possible to create

Box 15.1 H₁-antihistamines and pruritus[1]

In a convenience sample of 23 patients with a chronic stable pruritic dermatosis (21 atopic eczema, 2 psoriasis), subjects were allocated (?sequentially) to receive either:

- Astemizole 10 mg daily ($n=6$)
- Terfenadine 600 mg t.d.s. ($n=6$)
- Trimeprazine 10 mg t.d.s. ($n=7$)
- Nitrazepam 10 mg nocte ($n=7$).

(Three patients were used twice; they received trimeprazine a week after failing to obtain any benefit with terfenadine.)

Astemizole was given for several weeks; the other preparations for 2 days. The results for the four drugs are shown pictorially in Fig. 15.1. Eye-ball analysis suggests that the low-sedative second-generation H₁-antihistamines are ineffective in these circumstances but that a sedative H₁-antihistamine and a benzodiazepine have both a subjective and an objective effect. Formal analysis confirms that the differences observed are statistically significant ($p < 0.05$).

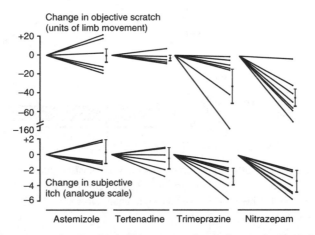

Fig. 15.1 Mean changes (and SE) in nocturnal scratch provoked by itching, measured in units of limb movement, and mean changes in subjective pruritus marked on a 10 cm line with median values. The results after stopping treatment are not given, but all patients returned to pretreatment levels. (From Krause and Shuster[1] 1983, with permission.)

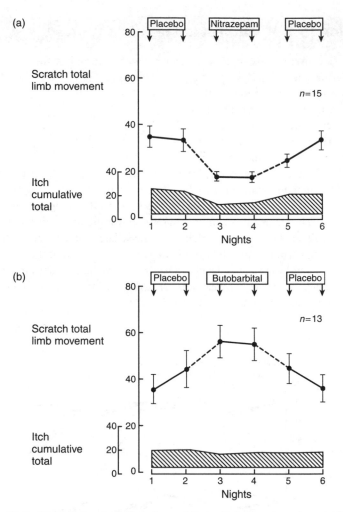

Fig. 15.2 Results of a study that showed that relief of nocturnal scratching by benzodiazepines (a) is not due to their hypnotic effect because a barbiturate (b) in comparable hypnotic dose makes scratching worse. (From Shuster[2] 1981, with permission.)

rational approaches with a good evidence base for managing pruritus in these situations (see Chapter 13). The main problem now is whether the relevant knowledge will be disseminated widely among clinicians and applied in practice. For example, in relation to uraemia, a physician's preference for drug therapy may mean that UVB phototherapy may be bypassed.[3] Given its potential for undesirable effects, unnecessary use of thalidomide could be unjustifiably harmful for some patients.[4, 5]

The discovery that an increase in opioidergic tone is the 'trigger' for pruritus in liver disease (see Chapter 5) may have implications for the scientific investigation of pruritus in pregnancy.[6] It is known that women who develop anicteric 'obstetric cholestasis' suffer from distressing pruritus.[7] This often affects mainly the soles of the feet and the palms of the hands (the classical early distribution in other forms of cholestasis). A recent study showed that, in a group of 10 women, pruritus developed between 2 and 20 weeks *before* the first biochemical evidence of abnormal liver function.[7]

Further, over a period of 2 weeks, colestyramine helped more than two-thirds of women with pregnancy pruritus,[8] even though plasma bile acid concentrations do not correlate well with the intensity of the pruritus.[9] However, as far as we know, no one has measured plasma endorphin concentrations in the women with pruritus or evaluated the effect of opioid antagonists.

The identification of a specific subset of unmyelinated C-fibres in peripheral nerves for the transmission of pruritus (see Chapter 2) has transformed the scientific study of pruritus. It is no longer possible to claim that pruritus and pain represent a sensory continuum, and it is only the intensity and/or the frequency of stimulation of peripheral nerves that determines whether a person experiences pruritus or pain. Although they share a common neuroanatomical pathway, pruritus and pain are distinct phenomena (Table 15.2).

As noted in Chapter 2, when pruritus is induced in volunteers by the intradermal application of histamine by injection or iontophoresis,

Table 15.2 Comparison of pain and pruritus

	Pain	**Pruritus**
Perception	Unpleasant	Generally unpleasant
Reflex response	Withdrawal	Scratch
Effect of NSAIDS	Generally relieves	Rarely relieves
Effect of opioids	Generally relieves	May cause
Scratching	Exacerbates	Relieves
Rubbing	Relieves	Relieves

functional positron emission tomography (fPET) demonstrates co-activation of several areas in the brain, including the cerebellum, with left-brain dominance.[10–12] The activation of multiple sites in the brain suggests that there is not a pruritus centre *per se* but, rather, a pruritus 'pattern generator' (see also Chapter 2). Co-activation of the motor area matches the clinical observation that pruritus is closely linked to a desire to scratch. Although the patterns of activation for pruritus and pain are similar, there are important differences, such as absence of detectable activation of the thalamus and somatosensory cortex in pruritus.

The present: clinical classification

A clinical classification of pruritus should help doctors to develop a more analytical approach in clinical evaluation and, in consequence, a more rational approach to treatment (see Chapter 13). Thus, it is pointless to apply topical drugs if the pruritus is neurogenic or neuropathic in origin. On the other hand, dry skin is generally an exacerbating factor in most patients with, for example, senile, hepatic, uraemic, or paraneoplastic pruritus. Thus skin care with an emollient should be considered basic treatment for all patients with pruritus. Uraemic pruritus is perhaps the best example of multifactorial pruritus, with several skin and several systemic factors interacting, possibly synergistically (see Chapter 6).

In relation to pruritus associated with the use of oral morphine in advanced cancer, even though the opioid effect *per se* is almost always central, other factors may well be involved and will influence management (Box 15.2).

The present: the AIDS pandemic

The HIV/AIDS pandemic in Sub-Saharan Africa, many parts of Asia, and several other countries has caused major health and socio-economic problems. Health services, already underresourced and overstretched, are faced with very difficult decisions about resource allocation. Thus, in South Africa, the Government has not sanctioned the routine use of antiretroviral drugs for people with AIDS. Apart from the adverse effect this must have on the course of AIDS and its outcome, it means that specific symptom relief will generally be all that can be offered.

In people who are HIV-positive, pruritus is common. It can be associated with dry skin and with several skin diseases, including eczema, psoriasis, and scabies, as well as with internal organ impairment or

Box 15.2 Pruritus and oral morphine

Likely to be multifactorial
• Dry skin
• High ambient temperature → vasodilatation and sweating
• Excipient in tablets?
• Morphine itself (central effect)
Approach to treatment
• Emollient
• Cool environment
• Drugs: diazepam 5 mg o.n. *and/or* ondansetron 8 mg b.d.
Note. Generally clears up spontaneously within 5–7 days.

neoplasia. Further, in those with a CD4 count below 300/µl, eosinophilic folliculitis may occur on the upper half of the body.[13] This is an intensely pruritic eruption with urticarial papules, plaques, or pustules associated with a raised plasma IgE concentration. Others who are HIV+ experience severe itching without an obvious rash or eosinophilia. It is possible that in some of these the cause may be neuropathic.[14] Sometimes, a non-steroidal anti-inflammatory drug (NSAID) is of benefit,[15] but frequently the pruritus remains intractable.

As always, 'necessity is the mother of invention' and, in the absence of antiretrovirals and with cost disincentives in relation to drugs such as fluconazole (for candidiasis), herbal remedies are being rediscovered or newly recognized,[16] though not as yet scientifically evaluated (Box 15.3).

Box 15.3 Topical herbal application for pruritus used in Southern Africa

Ingredients:
• Centella asiatica
• Bulbinella natalensis
• Bulbinella frutescens
• Lippia javanica
If associated with scabies or ringworm, add
• Flowers of sulphur

The future

Despite the need for effective remedies for pruritus, the likelihood that the pharmaceutical industry will invest billions of dollars in the search for effective non-sedative centrally acting antipruitics is surely zero. Given the relatively small numbers involved, such a project would not be commercially viable. This means that effective drug treatment for pruritus will always be a 'spin-off' from a drug developed and licensed for some other condition. Clinical interest in a drug is likely to be aroused as much by serendipity or coincidence as by considered pharmacological judgement.

Thus, pruritus is likely to remain a Cinderella symptom. However, we can hope that clinicians will take this relatively neglected symptom under their wing, and show determination and imagination in providing physical relief and psychological support for those who suffer from chronic pruritus associated with an underlying incurable condition.

References

1. Krause L, Shuster S. (1983). Mechanism of action of antipruritic drugs. *Br Med J (Clin Res Ed)* **287**:1199–200.

2. Shuster S. (1981). Reason and the itch. *Proc Royal Institution Great Britain* **53**: 136–63.

3. Szepietowski JC, Sikora M, Kusztal M, Salomon J, Magott M, Szepietowski T. (2002). Uremic pruritus: a clinical study of maintenance hemodialysis patients. *J Dermatol* **29**:621–7.

4. Ochonisky S, Verroust J, Bastuji-Garin S, Gherardi R, Revuz J. (1994). Thalidomide neuropathy incidence and clinico-electrophysiologic findings in 42 patients. *Arch Dermatol* **130**:66–9.

5. Fullerton PM, O'Sullivan DJ. (1968). Thalidomide neuropathy: a clinical electrophysiological, and histological follow-up study. *J Neurol Neurosurg Psychiatry* **31**:543–51.

6. Roger D, Vaillant L, Fignon A, *et al.* (1994). Specific pruritic diseases of pregnancy: a prospective-study of 3192 pregnant-women. *Arch Dermatol* **130**: 734–9.

7. Kenyon AP, Piercy CN, Girling J, Williamson C, Tribe RM, Shennan AH. (2001). Pruritus may precede abnormal liver function tests in pregnant women with obstetric cholestasis: a longitudinal analysis. *Brit J Obstet Gynaecol* **108**:1190–2.

8. Rampone A, Rampone B, Tirabasso S, Capuano I, Vozza G, Vozza A, Rampone N. (2002). Prurigo gestationis. *Journal of the European Academy of Dermatology and Venerology* **16**:411–27.

9. Jones EA, Bergasa NV. (1999). The pruritus of cholestasis. *Hepatology* **29**:1003–6.

10. Hsieh JC, Hägermark O, Stahle-Backdahl M, *et al.* (1994). Urge to scratch represented in the human cerebral cortex during itch. *J Neurophysiol* **72**:3004–8.

11. Darsow U, Drzezga A, Frisch M, *et al.* (2000). Processing of histamine-induced itch in the human cerebral cortex: a correlation analysis with dermal reactions. *J Invest Dermatol* **115**:1029–33.

12. Drzezga A, Darsow U, Treede RD, *et al.* (2001). Central activation by histamine-induced itch: analogies to pain processing: a correlational analysis of O-15 H_2O positron emission tomography studies. *Pain* **92**:295–305.

13. Rodwell GE, Berger TG. (2000). Pruritus and cutaneous inflammatory conditions in HIV disease. *Clin Dermatol* **18**:479–84.

14. Yosipovitch G, Greaves MW, Schmelz M. (2003). Itch. *Lancet* **361**:690–4.

15. Smith KJ, Skelton HG, Yeager J, Lee RB, Wagner KF. (1997). Pruritus in HIV-1 disease: therapy with drugs which may modulate the pattern of immune dysregulation. *Dermatology* **195**:353–8.

16. Miller MJ, Vergnolle N, McKnight W, *et al.* (2001). Inhibition of neurogenic inflammation by the Amazonian herbal medicine sangre de grado. *J Invest Dermatol* **117**:725–30.

Index